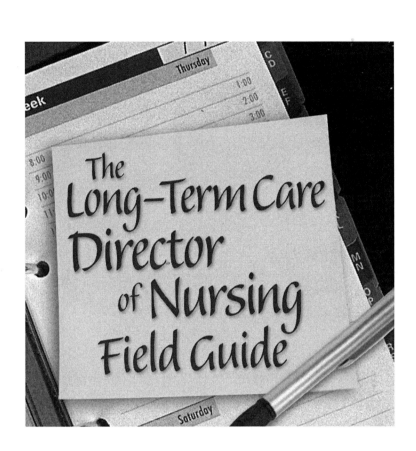

The
Long–Term Care
Director
of Nursing
Field Guide

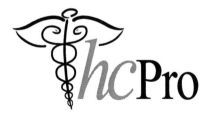

The Long-Term Care Director of Nursing Field Guide by HCPro, Inc.

Copyright © 2008 HCPro, Inc.

All rights reserved. Printed in the United States of America.   5   4   3   2   1

ISBN 978-1-60146-147-6

HCPro, Inc., provides information resources for the healthcare industry.

HCPro, Inc., is not affiliated in any way with The Joint Commission, which owns the JCAHO and Joint Commission trademarks.

Jo Walters, RNC, BC Gerontological Nurse, Reviewer

Adrienne Trivers, Managing Editor

Elizabeth Petersen, Executive Editor

Emily Sheahan, Group Publisher

Claire Cloutier, Production Manager

Jackie Diehl Singer, Graphic Artist

Patrick Campagnone, Cover Designer

Jean St. Pierre, Director of Operations

Liza Banks, Proofreader

Darren Kelly, Books Production Supervisor

Susan Darbyshire, Art Director

Paul Singer, Layout Artist

Advice given is general. Readers should consult professional counsel for specific legal, ethical, or clinical questions.

Arrangements can be made for quantity discounts. For more information, contact:

HCPro, Inc.
P.O. Box 1168
Marblehead, MA 01945
Telephone: 800/650-6787 or 781/639-1872
Fax: 781/639-2982
E-mail: *customerservice@hcpro.com*

Visit HCPro at its World Wide Web sites:
www.hcpro.com and *www.hcmarketplace.com*

4/2008

21390

CONTENTS

Contents

FOREWORD

Having been a director of nursing (DON) for over thirty years, one of my biggest complaints was the lack of reference materials geared to help me do my job. No one had put together a comprehensive guide on employee issues, leadership, successful orientation for the newly hired employee, conflict management, risk management, benchmarking, and delegation, to name a few among other issues.

I have always said that DONs need a bit of attention deficit disorder to do a great job. If we concentrate on any one area for too long, twenty more issues would have passed us by. DONs have dozens of issues and crises coming at them at once. We need to learn delegations and documentation to survive—After all we are endangered species, aren't we?

I think this book will be the DON's bible. It brings together many pieces of information that is needed to do a great job. For new DONs, it will also be a great learning tool. Seasoned DONs will also benefit by brushing up on areas that may not be our favorite thing to do. No one person can be an expert at everything, but with this book by your side, it will definitely enhance what you know about and what you are able to do well!

For those who are not DONs, this book will also be a great resource, and perhaps even serve as a stepping stone to prepare nurses who want to advance to become a supervisor, nurse manager, association of director of nursing, clinical care coordinator, or wellness nurse! It is written well and whether you work in assisted living, skilled care, adult day care, or at a rehab short stay facility, this reference will help you. We all have the same situations in different areas of work, and I am sure you will not regret purchasing this wonderful resource!

Sherrie Dornberger, RNC, CDONA, FACDONA
National Association of Directors of Nursing Administration
President

CHAPTER 1

Successful orientation of the newly hired manager

In your position, you hire many department managers and hope that they will accomplish great things for your organization. You have visions that their performance and skills will ease your workload and that they will bring ideas that renew and motivate staff—and, of course, that they will improve resident care.

As an administrative representative, your job is to improve the delivery of resident care in a fiscally sound and safe environment. The new manager you've hired has also been charged with this task. Sounds like quite a load to place on a brand-new hire, doesn't it? But you think to yourself, "That's what I hired this person for!" Several months or even a year may have passed since you last had a manager in that area, or maybe an interim manager has been filling the role. In some scenarios, you yourself have had to perform the responsibilities of the vacant manager along with your own duties. You sigh with great relief now that someone else will be handling the issues of that department.

First questions to ask yourself

Handing the baton to new managers may feel like a ton of weight lifting off your shoulders. You are more than ready to let them work their magic. But when this state of euphoria lifts, you will see that you have to rethink your perceptions of newly hired managers. This is not the time to set them loose without considering the following:

- Who will be orienting them?

- What is included in the orientation process for new managers at your organization?

- Have you verified their abilities to meet all aspects of the job description, or are you assuming that if they need help, they will ask?

- Is this the first management position for any new hire? If so, what training/support systems have you put into place for him or her?

Organizations invest a lot of time, money, and effort in orienting clinical staff. We know that such orientation improves staff performance, increases retention, promotes patient safety, and fulfills regulatory requirements. Why then do we treat newly hired managers differently? You have just spent a good deal of money, time, and effort to find them. You did background checks, contacted references, interviewed and reinterviewed them, and then hoped and prayed that they would accept your offer. How can you justify letting them go for it without a proper orientation after you exhausted all of those resources to find them?

Making excuses about lacking the time, funds, or resources to orient managers is not an acceptable practice. The absence of a comprehensive orientation process sends the following messages to new managers:

- The organization promised lots of things, but it won't deliver

- Lack of trust in the organization in the early onset of employment

- The organization sets unrealistic expectations

- This is why the previous manager left

Your role and position allow you to be the pivotal resource in new managers' success. Common obstacles to this success include the following:

- Your unrealistic expectations of them

- The absence of both a formal orientation process and the time to complete it

- The lack of a transition period (i.e., everything is dumped in new hires' laps from day one)

- Misconceptions regarding the role of the administrative person to whom new managers report

Designing an effective process

The administrative team needs to agree on the importance of a formal orientation program for managers, beyond the standard orientation for all employees. Look beyond the fire codes, employee handbook, and name badges to reach for another level. If you want new hires to manage and lead their departments effectively, give them the tools and resources they need to do so.

In putting together your formal orientation program for managers, consider the following:

- **Interview recent hires**—Survey your most recently hired managers and ask them questions about their orientation experiences. Explain what you are trying to improve and ask for their suggestions on how to do it.

- **Bring together "experts"**—Consider asking a seasoned manager, a member of the educational services department, or a human resources representative to lead the orientation process for the new managers.

- **Start building a library**—Begin collecting management resources that would benefit all of your departmental managers. This library can be located in your office, in the education office, or wherever new and experienced managers can access it regularly. Managers should be required to sign books in and out. Resources in your library should include:

  - Relevant journals, such as *Nursing Management*

  - Texts on leadership and coaching

  - Texts that are fun to read and that teach leadership principles at the same time (e.g., *Give 'em The Pickle*, by Robert Farrell)

  - Texts related to customer service

  - References about regulatory agencies

  - Web sites

  - Books with motivational quotes (for use on memos, in meetings, etc.)

As you develop this orientation process, managers in the organization who are not newly hired are going to see that they have missed out on something. Take this opportunity to examine your role in ongoing training for the midlevel management team as well. For example, areas of the orientation that cover skills like fiscal management may prove helpful to a manager who has been with you for two years. Open such sessions to your entire management team to promote the peer-group concept, help build the team, and provide consistency in management practices.

Essential elements of this orientation program include the following:

- An orientation process defined in writing, complete with schedule

- Time allotted (three to five shifts) for managers to orient themselves to being staff-level people in the departments for which they are responsible

- Clarification of your role and availability

- Making managers feel welcome from day one (e.g., avoiding responding to them as though their requests are tying you up)

- Setting only realistic expectations

- A resource library that is expanded on an ongoing basis

- Peer mentors with clear, well-defined (in writing) roles for each new manager

Use the template spreadsheets in this kit to assist you in outlining the orientation and schedule for new hires. Consider the qualifications and certifications required by the job description, and ask yourself, "How have I validated that they are competent in these areas?" Telling you during the interview that they are comfortable calculating full time equivalents (FTEs), working a budget plan, and understanding standards is one thing. Showing they can perform and apply this knowledge is another. Don't put yourself in a position where three weeks prior to the annual budget process you learn that this manager knows nothing about budgets or reading electronic financial sheets.

Uncover early in the orientation process those areas for which they will need your support or a referral to an appropriate person in the organization. Some key people to consider including in this orientation training are the department managers from:

- Materials management

- Nutrition services

- Fiscal services

- Human resources

- The employee assistance program

- Risk management

- Quality improvement

Also consider including a Joint Commission resource person.

The best way to initiate interaction with such people is simply to give the new hires copies of the organizational phone directory and highlight the departments you want them to call. Tell them to schedule some time with these department heads as part of their orientation—and before you send them off, be sure both parties know what you expect them to accomplish.

For example, when materials management meets with the new hires, you may want them to explain the following:

- How to complete a purchase requisition

- Who needs to sign requisitions and when an additional signature is required

- Current concerns related to the materials management department

- What capital purchase items are

- How to request special orders

When the new hires are going through this process (and, for that matter, all areas of the orientation), support them in taking the time to do these things before getting involved in the other areas of their job descriptions. You have waited this long to hire the person—one more week is not going to change anything. Inform staff and other department managers that new hires will be in orientation and that they will not be handed the job responsibilities until orientation is completed. Let whoever has been handling things in the absence of a manager continue to do so for one more week. This one decision alone will send a very important message to all of your midlevel managers: Administration appreciates them and realizes that they need time for training and information to do their jobs well. Now there is a great retention tool!

Orientation topics

Here are some steps to guide your orientation in conjunction with the templates located on this CD-ROM.

1. Organizational chart

Use this as a tool to:

- Identify where the new managers fit in

- Identify whom you report to

- Identify key administrative people with whom you would like new managers to schedule time

- Clarify to whom you expect new managers to go as a resource in your absence

2. Manager orientation templates

Review these templates and make changes appropriate to the managers' positions. Give copies to new hires and clarify your expectations in relation to their orientation processes. Set a target date for completion, and be sure to include a final copy in their personnel records.

3. Competency validations

If their roles include direct patient care, ensure that new hires have completed the competency requirements that a clinical staff person would have to demonstrate.

4. Introduce them to their mentors

Assign each hire to a mentor from his or her peer group. The selection of this person will play a great role in the transition process for the new manager. Meet with the two of them together to discuss and clarify your expectations.

5. Job description

Ask managers to closely review their job descriptions and, as they go through their first 90 days of employment, to identify areas that need changes or additions.

6. Clarifying your expectations

Not everything will be spelled out in the job description, and you shouldn't leave new hires to make assumptions about what is expected of them. Therefore, be sure to include the following in your initial discussions:

- Hours you expect them in the building/on campus

- Their availability to the department on weekends, holidays, evenings, and nights

- Their responsibility, if any, to cover staffing holes related to direct patient care

- How often you want them to schedule time with you and the best days/time to do so

- Your leadership style and how they can expect direction from you

7. Preparing the new managers' offices

Don't underestimate the welcome inherent in delegating to a secretary the job of setting up the new hires' offices and supplying them with the basic essentials. Your new managers should not have to spend their first days ordering staplers.

8. Communications

Explain the most productive method of communicating with you. It may be a combination of voice mail and e-mail. Maybe you prefer to read your e-mail only once a day, or maybe written notes and memos work better for you. Whatever your preference, share with managers the most effective and efficient way to communicate with you.

You may also elect to set up a once-a-week standing meeting date. If you do, help the managers to make the most of this time by discussing how to prepare for the meeting and what to bring to it. Items to consider asking your managers to arrive with include:

- Staffing sheets

- Budget reports

- Incident report follow-ups

- A list of questions they have compiled over the week

- Details about any obstacles that are interfering with their ability to do their jobs

9. Departmental priorities

Outline for managers what you perceive to be the priority needs for their departments. Discuss current issues related to resident care, staff performance, or risk management. Whether they are new to management or not, the three to five shifts they spend having a staff person orient them will provide them with more insight into the needs of the department than anything else could. This time also gives staff an opportunity to see their manager demonstrate competency and to get out there among the troops.

10. Regulatory agencies

Share with new hires any pending scheduled compliance reviews by the Joint Commision, state health department, etc. Determine their comfort level with their accountability to regulatory compliance organizations. If their previous job was held in another state, they may be unfamiliar with the standards in yours.

11. Physician issues

Don't let gossip be their only source of information about current physician issues. Part of your role is to help define their professional reality, and you accomplish this goal when you bring them up to date on nursing staff issues and concerns that the organization is currently facing. Also, provide an opportunity for managers to meet with the medical directors responsible for their departments. Share with them how the nursing staff committee process works in your organization. You can always defer this discussion to their mentors, if you feel it is appropriate to do so.

12. Payroll

Identify when you expect new managers to take over the payroll process. Provide adequate training time and support before handing over this responsibility—the last thing you want is to have payroll errors occur and have staff perceive the errors as the result of the new manager's incompetence.

13. Information systems (IS)

Nothing is more frustrating for new managers than wishing they could get ahold of some statistics that would help them in a process and simply not being able to find them—when everyone else knows where the statistics are. Part of the orientation process should include time with IS to share with managers what data is available and how to request it. Confirm during the first day of hire that new managers receive passwords to access anything related to IS, payroll, time clocks, etc.

14. Committee responsibilities

Outline the committees in which managers will need to participate, along with a schedule of when and where the meetings are held.

People working in healthcare management know very well the stressors, long hours, neverending fiscal challenges, etc., that welcome managers each day. With this in mind, consider the following:

- Have new hires recently relocated to accept this job? If so, ask whether they need any resources related to school for their children, places of worship, etc. Better yet, surprise them with an appointment with a representative of the local chamber of commerce, who has ready for them a local phone book, list of community resources, etc. Did they relocate without any family or support? If so, encourage a member of their peer group to join you and the new manager for dinner one evening during their first week.

- Realize that stress takes a physical and emotional toll, and beginning any new job is stressful. Just because you have chosen to work 14-hour days, five days a week doesn't justify laying that expectation on new managers.

- Are the managers going to be in school part-time to attain a degree required by the job description? If so, clarify your expectations and work together to balance school and work schedules.

Your ability to demonstrate effective leadership practices will be a springboard for all the managers on your team. When you begin the orientation process by demonstrating these practices through a formal orientation program, new managers will feel relieved to report to someone who understands their needs and desires for direction but who is also flexible enough to allow them to demonstrate their competencies in some areas that may not require as much of your time and attention.

In the book *Success is a Choice,* author Rick Pitino offers key points related to establishing good habits for success. Your good habits and practices in a leadership role define who you are and who the new managers may become.

"Ninety percent of the time, first impressions are the ones that last. Don't force people to require a second meeting to find out who you are." —Rick Pitino

Leadership

What is leadership?

Simply stated, leadership is the act of getting things done through other people. Doing so is not always simple—in fact, author Max Dupree believes that leadership is an art. He defines it as "liberating people to do what is required of them in the most effective and humane way possible." Further, leadership is different than management in that:

- Management focuses on efficiency (i.e., "Doing things right")

- Leadership focuses on effectiveness (i.e., "Doing the right things")

- Management is about getting things done

- Leadership focuses on what needs to be done and why

- Management deals with systems and structures

- Leadership is about relationships and engagement with people

- Management stresses consistency and control

- Leadership requires creativity, innovation, and "out-of-the-box" thinking

- Managers are concerned about results and the bottom line

- Leaders see the need to look over the horizon and have a vision

Stephen Covey summarizes these thoughts by explaining that managers focus on climbing the ladder in an efficient manner and leaders are concerned about the ladder being up against the right wall.

In the changing world of healthcare, there is clearly a need for both. The question is not "Am I a leader or a manager?" but rather "How do I develop both dimensions in my role as I work with staff on a daily basis?"

Qualities of effective leaders

Successful leadership is dependent on one's ability to:

- Inspire confidence

- Show personal interest

- Produce results and quality outcomes

- Inspire, gather, and use employees' ideas

- Lead rather than "boss"

- Foster teamwork and a sense of community

- Show kindness without being considered "easy"

- Coach staff to reach their potential

- Be a role model for balancing work and home

- Delegate properly

- Demonstrate self-confidence without being "cocky"

- Make hard decisions when needed

Successful leaders also share characteristics of emotional maturity (sometimes defined as an emotional quotient, or EQ), which set them apart. This emotional maturity is so important that many organizations include characteristics of it in the list of qualifications for a leadership or management role. They include the following:

- Self awareness—an awareness and respect for your gut feeling. This characteristic allows you to use emotions as sources of insight about yourself, others, and situations.

- Mood management—a proficiency in expressing feelings appropriately and controlling impulses.

- Self-starter—an innate drive to achieve, motivated internally by creative energy.

- Empathy—an ability to thoughtfully consider another's feelings (i.e., understand what makes them tick).

- People skills—an ability to manage relationships and bridge differences.

Emotional intelligence for leaders and managers is analogous to critical thinking skills for staff: it provides a key measure of success in the role. If you are interested in developing your own emotional intelligence, consider the following suggestions:

- Get feedback from your peers by asking these questions:

    - In a sentence, how do you see me?

    - If you could change one thing about me, what would it be?

    - If I were to keep doing one thing I'm doing, what should it be?

    - What is your definition of an effective leader?

- Stay in touch. Take time for small talk with staff, especially with your quieter members.

- Be ruthlessly honest with yourself rather than blaming others.

- Remove barriers. Ask the staff about barriers they encounter in trying to get their work done and then follow up on those that you can impact.

- Avoid "us and them" or "win–lose" thinking—the goal is collaboration, not polarization.

Situational leadership

Everyone agrees that effective leadership is vital to a group's success. But trying to reach a consensus about which behaviors constitute effective leadership is not so easy. This lack of agreement suggests that, depending on the situation, a wide range of leadership behaviors can be effective.

Situational leaders change their leadership styles depending on the situation and person with whom they are working. Three skills are involved in being a situational leader:

- Diagnosing: Pinpoint the needs of the people with whom you work.

- Flexibility: Use a variety of leadership styles.

- Partnering: Come to some agreements with staff about the leadership style they need from you.

Four basic leadership styles

For a long time, people thought there were only two leadership styles—autocratic and democratic. In fact, people used to shout at each other from these two extremes, insisting that one style was better than the other. Democratic managers were accused of being too soft and easy, while their autocratic counterparts were often called too tough and domineering. Today's manager, however, is flexible and is able to use all four of the leadership styles described below.

Leadership and staff empowerment

For many years, leaders were believed to be effective because of personality or personal charisma. This was called the "trait theory" of leadership, and it was not until the Ohio State management and leadership studies by Paul Hersey and Ken Blanchard in the late 1960s that this conventional wisdom was debunked. Through their research, they found effective leaders had a talent for aligning the style they used with the particular needs of the person or group with whom they were dealing. This approach became known as "situational leadership," reflecting that the leader varies his or her style and uses "different strokes for different folks."

To use this approach effectively, learn to diagnose which style is needed when and become comfortable moving between four different styles depending on the situation. Over the course of usually three to five years, the staff with whom you are working should progress from requiring a directing style (e.g., orientation) to a coaching style (e.g., they are competent and developing talents) to a more independent phase in which you support their decisions and can finally delegate, knowing that you can trust their judgment.

Because staff gain authority as they develop, leaders, in a sense, work themselves out of a job. It has often been said that "the effectiveness of a leader is measured by what happens in his or her absence." The four basic leadership styles leaders can use to develop staff are described in more detail below.

1. Directing—In this style, the leader provides specific direction and closely monitors the accomplishment of tasks. Communication is largely one-way: You tell staff what, when, where, and how to do something, and then you closely monitor their performance on the problem or task. You explain what the goal is and what a good job looks like, and you also lay out a step-by-step plan for meeting that goal. Essentially,

you solve the problem. You make the decisions and the person carries out your ideas. A directing style is appropriate:

- When a decision has to be made quickly and the stakes are high

- For inexperienced people who you think have the potential to be self-directive

- For someone who has some skills but doesn't know the organization (e.g., the past history, established protocols, or political implications of a situation)

Usually, staff will not resent direction and close supervision when they are first learning a task. Most people are enthusiastic beginners. They are ready for any help you can give them because they want to perform well.

2. Coaching—As the staff member or group begins to understand the expectations and move through the novice phase in development of skills and abilities, you will need to change to two-way communication with a coaching style. Good coaches bring out the best in people by helping them see their talents and abilities and the value they add to the team. They also are adept at pointing out the "rough edges" that need more work or the skills that need to be added to the basic ones they acquired in the first year of employment. Because staff are moving from being a novice to functioning in an independently competent manner, it is appropriate to involve them in the process with questions like, "What can I do to make you more effective?"

Many managers find this phase in the staff development process to be very rewarding as they watch staff blossom in their roles and grow in their senses of self-esteem. The coaching style works best with:

- Staff that want to develop a particular interest in technical skills or competence in a new process, such as discharge planning

- A group that has a sense of what it wants to accomplish but needs help learning to manage a meeting or reach consensus

- Employees who have transferred from another department or job and have the basic skills but need the finer points of their new roles explained

3. Supporting—As staff accept more responsibility for and become proficient in their roles, the leader shares with them the decision-making and problem-solving

responsibilities and supports them in applying their ideas. The leader can be much less directive in this role due to the proficiency of the person or group, and, in a sense, it becomes the leader's job not to give answers but to ask the right questions. For example, you might say, "Tell me what needs to happen because you are the ones who have to make this work," or, "I need to know the pros and cons of this policy as we have developed it, so let me know what you think and then we can get it finalized."

Supporting style works best with:

- Staff who are two or three years into the job and have developed their ideas about what needs to be done to improve the work environment

- Experienced staff who are brought together on a short-term task force that needs to produce results

- Staff who have transferred from another facility (who have demonstrated proficiency in the role) and want to implement some ideas that worked in their earlier employment

4. Delegating—In this style, the leader turns over the responsibility for day-to-day decision-making and problem solving to staff. This style offers the most latitude for authority in decisions and autonomy. Delegating is appropriate for people who are self-reliant achievers—people who are competent and committed and who therefore do not need much direction. They are also able to provide their own support. For example, top performers do not need much supervision or praise as long as they know how well they are doing. Leaders using this style present the problem and then get out of the way as staff develop a solution. Delegating works best with:

- Seasoned experts who are ready for "job enrichment," so they can stay enthusiastic and invested in their role and make a contribution

- Issues like staff scheduling, because staff know what needs to happen and are able to make it happen using guidelines agreed upon by the group

- Task forces that have implemented a process and need to fine-tune it or maintain and update its structure

Identifying the best leadership style for the situation

There is no best way to influence others. The right choice of leadership style depends on your ability to determine whether your staff have all the skills and experience they need to do the job they are assigned and your sense of whether they want to or believe they can do it.

Assess readiness as determined by the level of competence and commitment the person or group brings to the job to be done. Taking the time to accurately diagnose how to best align leadership style with staff needs is the characteristic feature of situational leadership. Leaders who fail to accurately assess these needs often rely on instinct, assumptions, or their own favorite styles and thereby miss the opportunity to really engage with their staff.

Micromanagement and being left to "sink or swim" are just two examples of the lack of alignment between a leader and follower(s). To increase the chances of aligning with the readiness of staff or the group, give thought to the concepts of competence and commitment, as they are equally important to accomplishing a task or being successful in a role.

Competence—Competence is a function of knowledge and skills, which can be gained from education, training, and experience. Competence is not another word for ability—people often use the word ability to mean potential, and they talk about "natural" ability to describe why some people seem to be able to learn certain skills easily. Competence, however, can develop with the appropriate direction and support. You are not born with competence—you learn it.

Commitment—Commitment is a combination of confidence and motivation. Confidence is a measure of a person's self-assuredness—a feeling of being able to do a task well without much supervision—and motivation is a person's interest in and enthusiasm for doing a task well. If employees have the competence and confidence to do a job but no motivation, they are not committed to it. Sometimes, for example, people lose motivation when they realize the task is going to be harder to complete than they thought.

When we examine the relationship between the four leadership styles, commitment, and competence, we find the following:

- Directing is for those who lack competence and, because of their insecurity, lack commitment (e.g., orientees or new grads in their first year of employment).

- Coaching is for those who are committed and not so insecure but need guidance, praise, and feedback to continue developing their competence (e.g., staff with 15–36 months on the job).

- Supporting is for those who are competent in that their skills are well-developed but who need support and guidance in trusting their own judgment and making decisions that build their self esteem (e.g., a proficient staff nurse who is chosen to chair a task force of her peers).

- Delegating is for those who have both competence and commitment. They are willing and able to work on a project by themselves and with little supervision or support.

Self-assessments

It is important for the leader to thoughtfully assess the style needed by a person or group, but it is also helpful to have the person or group use these ideas to assess themselves and ask for the style they need from the leader.

This framework can shed light on what staff need in terms of guidance and support. They may report to a director who naturally prefers a delegating style. However, if they are new in the management role, the director will need to use more of a directing style with them. If they are seasoned expert managers and are reporting to a director who is new, they may find themselves micromanaged as the director sorts out how much guidance they need. Candid and honest discussions about such alignments can be instrumental in everyone's overall effectiveness. Allow situational leadership to provide a framework for these important conversations.

Case Study: Applying leadership styles to problem solving

A seasoned employee has approached you with concerns about a new medication adminis-tration policy. In the past, this employee has been reluctant to participate in problem-solving processes. You identify this as an opportunity to use a combination of the leadership styles you learned in this module: directing, coaching, supporting, and delegating.

Consider this response: "You have identified a real potential problem with this new policy. It is good that you brought it to my attention—thank you so much. I understand the pharmacy committee is meeting Wednesday to address concerns that have been voiced by staff, and it would be very beneficial for them to hear your perspective. Since you are already sched-uled for that day and the meeting is at 10 a.m., I will cover your assignment for you while you attend. If you need any references or resources to support your ideas, please feel free to use any of the materials on my bookshelf or let me know if I can be of any help. Thanks again for bringing this to my attention. It will be interesting to see the outcome of the meeting, won't it?"

Recommended reading

1. Bozell, Jeanna. A Nurse Leaders's Instruction Book-Ultimate Resource for Retaining Staff. Muncie, Indi-ana: Nurse Quest, 2003.

2. Dupree, Max. Leadership is an Art. New York: Doubleday Publishing, 1989.

3. Goleman, Daniel. Working with Emotional Intelligence. New York: Bantam Books, 2000.

4. Hersey, Paul, Ken Blanchard and Dewey Johnson. Management of Organizational Behavior 8th Edition. Upper Saddle River, NJ: Prentice-Hall, 2001.

5. Kouzes, James and Barry Posner. Credibility: How Leaders Gain and Lose It, Why People Demand It. San Francisco: Jossey-Bass, 1993.

6. Kouzes, James and Barry Posner. The Leadership Challenge. San Francisco: Jossey-Bass, 1990.

7. Lencioni, Patrick. The Five Dysfunctions of a Team. San Francisco: Jossey-Bass, 2002.

8. Manion, Jo. From Management to Leadership. Chicago: AHA Press, 1998.

Communication

An essential skill set for effective managers is communicating clearly and honestly both on a one-to-one basis and in groups. Staff value managers who communicate with them in an adult manner rather than in a parent-child or boss-to-subordinate style. When the manager is truthful and makes every effort to share information, staff know they can ask questions or check out rumors with their manager, and as decisions are made, staff feel in-the-loop and "on the same page" as their manager. Such open, trusting communication is the foundation of teamwork and high-quality resident care. But reaching this goal is not necessarily easy or simple for any of the following reasons:

We only hear what we expect to hear. What we hear or understand when someone speaks to us is largely shaped by our own experience and background. Instead of hearing what people tell us, we hear what our minds tell us has been said—and the two may be the same or they may be very different.

We all tend to have preconceived ideas of what people mean. When we hear something new, we tend to identify it with something similar that we have experienced in the past. In addition, most of us resist change. We tend to reject new ideas, particularly if they conflict with what we already believe. In many ways, our communications-receiving apparatus works like a filter: when we read a paper or listen to a political speech, we tend to note only those things that confirm our present beliefs and ignore anything that conflicts.

The perceptions of the source and recipient are different. The group with which we identify ourselves tends to shape our interpretation of the communications we receive. Generation X employees, for instance, are not likely to volunteer for significant amounts of overtime because they place a high value on personal balance and a life outside of work. Managers often get more volunteers from other staff members (e.g., Generation Y or baby boomers), who tend to be more team-minded.

We evaluate the source rather than the message. It is extremely difficult for us to separate what we hear from our feelings about the person who says it. Not only do receivers evaluate what they hear in terms of their own backgrounds and experiences, they also take the senders into account. How reliable are they as sources of information? Do they have an axe to grind? Are they agitators? Feelings about messengers can interfere with our ability to hear their messages.

Our emotional state affects what we hear. When we are insecure, worried, or fearful, what we hear and see seems more threatening than it does when we are secure and at peace with the world. Rumors may fly when unexpected or unexplained changes occur. Statements and actions that under less trying circumstances would have passed unnoticed become grounds for fear. By the same token, when we are angry or depressed, we tend to reject out of hand what might otherwise seem like a reasonable request or a good idea. Our negativity influences what we see and hear.

Ways to improve your communication

- Get to know your staff—Who are your introverts (i.e., staff that need time to process information internally)? Who are your extroverts (i.e., staff who need to process information by talking about it so they can clarify what they think as they talk)? Consider gender differences in learning style: Men usually like to cut to the chase, and women tend to prefer stories and examples.

- Hold routine staff meetings—Preferably held on the same day each month, the staff meeting provides an opportunity for the manager to update staff on pertinent information and recognize them for their contributions. It is also a time for task forces and unit councils to report on their activities so that the right hand knows what the left hand is doing. A group setting is the perfect time for managers to ask key questions, such as, "What would it look like if we really believed in teamwork?" Staff meetings also provide an ideal time for managers to explain challenges (i.e., sell the problem) and to have staff come up with solutions they would like to see implemented.

- Establish expectations or team agreements—The expectations you have for your staff should answer the following question: "What do I need from you and what do you need from me in order for us to work well together?" These expectations can be updated quarterly and used to set behavior standards or group norms.

You should expect that staff:

- Keep you informed of any situation that might escalate

- Talk out differences with each other rather than acting them out

- Speak to you first if they have a problem with you

The staff may expect that you:

- Keep them informed of decisions impacting the unit

- Support their efforts to grow and develop by offering timely feedback

- Advocate for them when dealing with disruptive physician behaviors

- Visually present progress on projects or key indicators to staff whenever possible— Charts, diagrams, and flow charts convey a great deal of information in a concise manner and often assist staff in focusing on issues or getting the big picture on phases of a change process.

- "Walk the talk"—Staff are more likely to get on board with needed changes if they see that managers hold themselves to the same behavior standards they have set for their staff. If managers ask staff to answer lights whether or not it is their patient, then staff expect to see managers answer lights when feasible. This is essential in developing a sense of trust and partnership between managers and staff, and it is a make-or-break factor in managers' credibility with their employees. A lack of credibility will derail managers' communication efforts.

- Routinely ask for feedback—Foster teamwork and a sense of community at work by asking staff for feedback on what's working or not working and what needs to be done differently. Staff should have the opportunity at least twice a year to evaluate the manager and offer suggestions for changes in what the manager is doing. Fostering an open-door policy and being approachable and available to staff on all shifts is critical in developing communication-driven teamwork.

- Tie either a communication book or an e-mail communication system to the job description—This clarifies staff responsibilities regarding the information contained in whichever communication system you chose to use. Staff may be asked to initial each page they review in the communication book, or they may be asked to be responsible to an e-mail system. Some staff will not do either, but you still hold them accountable for the information contained in these communications.

"Managing up"

Just as maintaining open, honest communication is essential for effective managers, it is equally important to manage the relationship you have with the person to whom you report. Keeping lines of communication open, having a shared sense of priorities, and fostering a collegial relationship provides you with a source of support and mentoring. In this regard, it is helpful to:

- Have routine, one-on-one meetings for one hour at least every two weeks. If you are new in your positions, consider doing this weekly for a period of time.

- Review priorities quarterly and discuss resources needed.

- Follow up on ongoing issues to ensure that deadlines are met.

- Ask for assistance as needed in removing organizational barriers or dealing with system issues involving other departments.

- Talk through or role-play situations in which coaching is needed for the manager's effectiveness.

Providing feedback to staff

In national surveys of the healthcare workplace, lack of recognition is an issue that often ranks in the top-10 issues that staff feel need manager's attention. All too often, managers focus on behavior problems with staff and fail to recognize those who are meeting or exceeding expectations on a regular basis. In this regard, a useful practice for managers is to routinely write thank you notes to the employees you observe doing a good job and send these notes to the employee's home. Although the suggestion is for this to be routine (i.e., two or three notes a week), it is important that the notes be sincere and specific about the behavior being referenced.

When constructive feedback is warranted, keep in mind the following tips:

- Be specific—Feedback is useful only when the person receiving it knows exactly what needs to change. Generalizing or being indirect can lead to mixed messages.

- Convey the impact of the behavior—Sharing your feelings about the impact of the behavior can be powerful in getting that person's attention. For example, say, "When you fail to attend staff meetings, I feel as though you don't want to be a part of our team, and we lose the insight and experience you have to offer."

- Use "I" statements, and keep them brief, so as not to lecture—Your correspondences should include statements that begin with the following:

  - "I feel . . . "

  - "I need for you to . . . "

  - "What I would rather have is . . . "

- Practice this approach at home and with friends to get comfortable being direct and honest, as opposed to using the "weasel language" managers sometimes use.

  - "It's not a big deal, but if you could just, sort of, try to do a little better, then maybe we could . . . "

The art of active listening

To quote George Bernard Shaw, "The greatest problem of communication is the illusion that it has been accomplished." All too often we fail to communicate by failing to listen. The ability to listen empathetically so that the person talking with you feels heard and understood is a valuable skill set for managers. Rather than just listening for a pause in the conversation so that you know when to begin talking, practice the art of active listening by doing the following:

- Take the time to probe and listen more. Doing so requires you use phrases like, "Tell me more," "What makes that so important to you," "For example," and "What else do I need to know?" Pay close attention to the added details to which these prompts lead.

- Nonverbally communicate that you are listening. Maintain eye contact, nod your head, etc.

- Listen to understand. Stephen Covey, a management guru, points out the value of "Seeking first to understand and then to be understood."

- Paraphrase or restate what you hear. You can initiate this technique with phrases like

"If I heard you correctly then . . . ", "I hear you saying that . . . ", "The situation then is . . ."

- Developing the art of listening takes time and practice, but the benefits of becoming a good listener are significant. Staff are more likely to listen to you if they find that you routinely listen to them—active listening is reciprocal. Additionally, when you take the time to actively listen, you may well see the situation differently and make other choices than you would have made by jumping to conclusions or reading into a situation.

- Recognize also that you need to act on the requests of your staff because the only way they know they have been heard is when something happens with what they said. Taking ownership for your part in resolving an issue or following up on a problem goes a long way in building your credibility as a manager.

- After your next conversation, test your ability to benefit from listening to it. Analyze and ask yourself the following:

  - What did I learn from the other person(s)?

  - What did I learn about the other person(s)?

  - Who did more talking?

  - Who did more listening?

  - Did anyone interrupt?

  - What questions should I have asked?

  - What questions should I have answered more thoroughly?

  - Was I absolutely certain I understood everything?

  - Did I ask for clarification?

  - Did I practice acknowledgement?

  - Did he or she practice acknowledgement?

  - Did anyone keep changing the subject?

  - Did anyone appear angry or sad?

  - Was everyone paying attention?

  - What will I do differently in my next conversation?

The ability to listen is a skill that can be improved with use. This skill can and will improve all your relationships.

Case Study: Reading nonverbal communication cues

Q Justin is in your office because when he worked yesterday, he had made a medication error and wants to talk to you about it. He repeatedly explains to you that he is not upset, and he says, "I just want to be sure that I am following that new policy for med errors." You also notice the following:

- Minimal eye contact

- Tearing up of his eyes

- Unwillingness to take a seat when you offer him one

What will be the key to effective communication in this situation?

A *Effective communication skills for the manager require the ability to identify nonverbal clues to guide the discussion. This knowledge will help direct your response, which might be the following: "Justin, I appreciate your coming by today to talk about the med error. I hear you say that you are not upset, but I see it differently. Your eyes are tearing, you won't look at me, and, knowing you to be the excellent nurse that you are, I believe you probably are upset. So go ahead and have a seat, and let's chat about the fact that you are human and you made a mistake." If you have made a med error yourself in the past, regardless of how long ago, this is the perfect time to share that experience with Justin.*

Recommended reading

1. Block, Peter. Stewardship: Choosing Service Over Self Interest. San Francisco: Barrett-Kohler, 1993.

2. Connors, Roger. The Oz Principle: Getting Results Through Accountability. Englewood Cliffs, NJ: Prentice Hall, 1994.

3. Covey, Stephen. The 7 Habits of Highly Effective People. New York: Simon and Schuster, 1989.

4. Hersey, Paul, Ken Blanchard, and Dewey Johnson. Management of Organizational Behavior 8th Edition. Upper Saddle River, NJ: Prentice-Hall, 2001.

CHAPTER 4

Building a budget

The budget cycle

A budget is a financial plan that outlines the resources an entity foresees using for a particular time period. The master budget encompasses all the departmental budgets. Based on the organization's strategic goals and vision, the master budget is the actual statement of projected revenues and expenditures for the entire hospital.

Developing a budget is an ongoing process. See the budget cycle in Figure 4.1 to better understand the order and process of the budget cycle.

FIGURE 4.1   **The budget cycle**

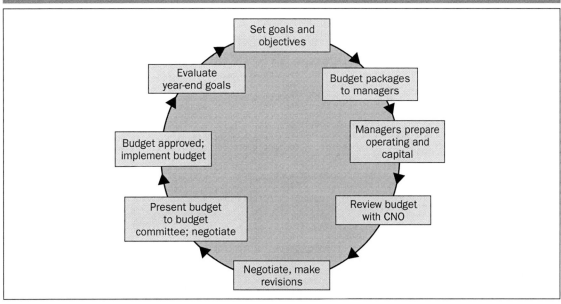

The budget cycle typically involves an environmental assessment that looks at trends in healthcare and in the facility as well as its competition. Once such assessments are made, the facility's goals and objectives are evaluated to determine whether any changes must be made. If changes must be made, goals are set based on the prior year's performance, trends in the marketplace, and assumptions about the future.

The organization's operational objectives are developed and approved by the administrative department. It is at this point that the formal budget packages—including instructions, projected units of service (UOS), and revenue for the unit—are put together and distributed to department managers. Expect to receive such a package approximately four to six months before the budget is due.

Next, you will prepare your budget. At this point, negotiations between the nurse manager and the chief nurse executive (CNE) or chief nursing officer (CNO), as well as any other departments, occur. Once the CNE approves your budget, you present it to the appropriate group(s), which usually consist of administration and the chief financial officer (CFO). The CFO will likely have questions the manager needs to address. Following the meeting with administration and the CFO, you must make the necessary adjustments to your budget. If there is an opportunity to re-present or appeal the budget, this is the time to do so. The budget is then approved, stamped, sealed, and ready to be implemented.

Finally, at the year's end, it is time to evaluate the annual budget. After doing so, you can determine what needs to be modified for next year's budget. Do this by tracking and trending activities and numbers throughout the year to develop a fair and reasonable budget for the following year.

In many facilities, the finance department and administration work together to develop a budget calendar. This calendar is distributed to all managers and helps keep everyone on the same page with their budgeting tasks for the upcoming year.

At the end of the budget cycle, the facility will create an operating budget that it must present to and get approved by the board of directors.

Controllable and uncontrollable expenses

You are responsible for managing the activities of your facility; therefore, you must know what you have control over. Typically, you control most of the activities in your facility that contribute to the budget. Such activities include staffing, skill mix, education, staff meetings, and orientation length. At the end of each month, you must explain to your supervisor any discrepancies in the numbers you budgeted. Internal accounting reports are usually given to managers. Such reports show the difference between the expected performance planned in the budget and the actual results.

Your responsibilities are as follows:

1. Controllable expenses

- Staffing

- Supplies

2. Uncontrollable expenses

- Revenue

- Patients' acuity levels and unit activity levels

- Types of benefits

Types of budgets

There are many types of budgets that you may be responsible for or for which you will make contributions.

Expense budget

Managers are typically involved in developing two types of budgets: operating and capital. The operating budget entails the facility's day-to-day plan for revenue and expenses. Most facilities generate expenses, which might include the following:

1. Personnel expenses

- Wages

- Salaries

- Benefits

- Overtime

- Orientation

- Education

2. Other expenses

- Supplies (medical and nonmedical)

- Minor equipment

- Linen

- Purchased services

- Maintenance

- Food

- Interdepartmental transfers

As you can see, expenses are broken down into two components: personnel and other expenses.

Personnel budget

The finance department or your supervisor will determine the projected budgeted revenue for your facility, and then expenses must be calculated. As mentioned earlier, the biggest expense is staff salaries. In fact, salaries often account for up to 75% of budgets. The personnel budget determines how much staff is needed to operate the facility 24 hours a day, 365 days a year.

Budgeted staff in nursing includes the following, and may include additional staff at your facility:

- Nurse manager

- Charge nurses

- Registered nurses (RNs)

- Licensed practical nurses (LPNs)

- Nursing assistants (NAs)

- Monitor technicians

- Orderlies

- Clerical staff

Budgeted staff in ancillary areas includes some of the following, and may include additional staff at your facility:

- Department manager

- Assistant managers (if applicable)

- Pharmacist

- Physical therapist

- Respiratory therapist

- Technicians

- Assistants

- Clerical staff

The personnel budget is typically a variable budget—the numbers rise and fall depending on the volume and complexity of cases. The opposite of the variable budget is the fixed budget, which remains constant. Some ancillary areas have fixed budgets, but others do not. A fixed budget means that the department has fixed staffing or does not flex staffing with volume fluctuations. Check with your supervisor or finance department to clarify the type of budget you are responsible for and what the expectations are of you managing it.

In both inpatient and outpatient areas, other line items may be fixed, regardless of the volume. For example, if you allot $200 per month for minor equipment, this amount stays the same regardless of the volume of patient cases.

Budgeting methods

Different organizations may have different budgeting practices. For instance, some facilities use computerized programs to develop their budgets, while others still calculate by hand. With some systems, nurse managers are handed a budget and asked to review, edit, and return it by a certain date; others are expected to perform the "zero-based budget method," or ZBB, requiring the manager to build a budget from scratch.

ZBB

ZBB is the most effective and widely used method for budgeting. It consists of calculating projected costs by line item from the bottom up. In other words, rather than looking at the budget history, the new budget is built upon calculated assumptions. By using this method, you can analyze data and consider alternatives rather than relying solely on the previous year's numbers. (Much of what is covered in the salary portion of expenses throughout this chapter resembles the ZBB method.) But let's look at other models.

Flat percentage increase

The flat percentage increase method begins with a predetermined percentage, which is provided to you. This percentage is then added to the current actual number to determine the budget number. For example, assume that for eight months salaries year-to-date (YTD) are $525,000. By figuring out the annualized number ($525,000 ÷ 8 months = $65,625 x 12 months = $787,500), you can then move to the next step. Multiply the annualized expense ($787,500) by the predetermined percentage (10%) to calculate next year's increase ($78,750). Add the increase to the annualized expense to reach the total expenses ($866,250) you can plan to pay for the next year.

Although this method is quick and easy, it does not take into consideration productivity, nor does it require analysis. It is important for you to look at the entire picture and learn from the previous year's experiences to produce a credible, realistic budget. Because of this, the ZBB method is most prominent in hospitals.

Computer budgeting software

Another way to calculate budgets is by using sophisticated computer software. Budgeting software has come a long way and is fairly user-friendly. Depending on the software, programs can be fairly expensive, so don't be discouraged if your hospital is not equipped with the software. The most important thing to remember is if your organization is willing to purchase such software, make sure your finance department approves it.

Constructing your budget

Personnel expenses

There are many steps related to determining personnel expenses for your budget. The rest of the chapter discusses 13 steps you can take to calculate these expenses.

Step #1: Gathering data

To prepare your unit's annual budget, at a minimum gather the following data regarding salary expenses:

Budgeted UOS or patient days

UOS projections may or may not include your input. Some facilities give managers the budgeted UOS and then assign them the responsibility of determining the needed personnel and other required resources based on those projections. Other facilities negotiate with managers to determine UOS. Information used to determine UOS includes the previous year's actual UOS, projections for the upcoming year, and other factors, such as changes in the facility's physical layout, new programs or physicians coming or leaving, and closing or opening of competing facilities.

If you are told that your UOS are "flat," this means that next year your facility's UOS is expected to remain the same. If you do not agree with the projected or budgeted UOS for your new budget, present data to validate your assumptions (e.g., historical data or information regarding new patient classification types). Present these data early in the budgeting process.

Budgeted hours per patient day (HPPD)

To figure salary expenses, you must know the HPPD—or standard of productive, direct-care hours. HPPD is determined in a manner similar to UOS. To figure HPPD, facilities will also look at benchmarks from national databases (e.g., those of HBSI International, Inc., or nursing associations) and compare the databases' data to the facility's operation figures. When comparing facilities, make sure what comprises the HPPD in other facilities is the same as in yours. For example, if your facility's HPPD includes orientation and education/training, don't compare your facility to another facility's that only looks at productive time. Think critically, and be willing to ask questions. Do not just accept these numbers from your finance department. In ancillary areas, the standard may be hours per visit, test, procedure, exam, or other.

For the purposes of calculating HPPD, assume the nursing unit budgeted 67,500 hours the previous year. By dividing the total budgeted hours (67,500) by the UOS (7,500), the HPPD comes to 9.0 (67,500 ÷ 7,500 = 9.0).

Average and unit average hourly rates

Some organizations do not give managers the HPPD but the total budgeted hours by job category, whereas others provide only a total salary dollar target and orders for the nurse manager not to be concerned with HPPD. When given the total budgeted hours by job category, determine the average hourly rate for the previous year. To do this, look at the total actual salary dollars for the previous year and divide that amount by the total hours worked. For example, if you paid $1,200,200 in productive salaries and used 65,700 total hours worked by staff, the average hourly rate for the previous year would be $18.27 ($1,200,000 ÷ 65,700 = $18.27).

Rather than breaking down the average hourly rates by job category, set a unit average hourly rate. Add together the hourly rates for each employee, and divide that total by the number of job categories. This number is determined by using the following equation:

(sum of hourly rates) ÷ number of job categories = unit average hourly rate

For example, if the average hourly rate for an RN is $25, for an LPN is $18, and for an NA is $9, then the unit average hourly rate equals $17.33 ([$25 + $18 + $9] ÷ 3 = $17.33). We will use this unit average hourly rate for future examples.

Skill mix

Another process you must become involved in is the skill mix breakdown. When determining this breakdown, take into consideration the type of nursing care model, the facility policy regarding use of LPNs and NAs, and patient acuity levels. In ancillary areas, the use of technicians or assistants would need to be considered. For the purposes of this book, use the following skill mix percentages: 75% RN, 10% LPN, and 15% NA.

Other considerations when calculating salary expenses

Productive and nonproductive hours

Salary expenses include productive hours (actual time worked or direct-care hours) and nonproductive (nonworked) hours. Nonproductive hours include orientation, education, vacation, sick time, holidays, etc. In preparing your budget, allocate required productive, or direct-care, hours. To determine productive hours, use the following equation: UOS x HPPD = total productive hours required.

For example, if the annual budgeted UOS is 7,500 and the budgeted HPPD is 9.0, then the total productive hours required is 67,500 (7,500 x 9.0 = 67,500).

Direct and indirect costs

Costs the facility incurs—and that you are responsible for—are called direct costs. Direct costs are those associated with the delivery of resident care. Some direct costs include salaries for

RNs, LPNs, NAs, orderlies, and monitor technicians. Other examples of direct costs include supplies, administration fees, and electricity bills.

Indirect costs are those assigned to the unit from other areas. They are costs that are necessary for, but do not directly relate to, the delivery of resident care. For example, services from the biomedical engineering department, or bio-med, fall under indirect costs. For instance, bio-med staff make routine inspections of nursing department equipment. Such maintenance costs are typically charged to the nursing department, because the service was for the unit where the resident received care; therefore, the bio-med department would not be charged.

Budget data

Review the budget data in Figure 4.2. It will be used throughout the chapter.

FIGURE 4.2   **Sample budget data**

(Unit has 26 bed capacity)		
UOS: 7,500		
HPPD: 9.0		
Average hourly rate:	RN:	$25/hour
	LPN:	$18/hour
	NA:	$ 9/hour
Unit average hourly rate:	$17.33	
Skill mix:	RN:	75%
	LPN:	10%
	NA:	15%

Step #2: Calculating ADC

Next determine your unit's budgeted average daily census (ADC). ADC is important because it helps you explain variances and project staffing. It is needed also for subsequent calculations throughout this chapter. See the following exercise to get a better understanding of how ADC is calculated.

Exercise

What is your ADC?

UOS ÷ 365 or 7,500 ÷ 365 = 20.55

What is your budgeted occupancy rate?

ADC = 20.55 per day ÷ 26 beds x 100% = 79%

There are 67,500 productive hours budgeted for providing care to the ADC. The ADC represents 20.55 residents per day for 365 days. Next determine who will provide resident care and how. Remember that not all staff work full-time; in fact, if you operate a 12-hour shift unit, each full-time employee will likely work 72 hours per pay period rather than the typical 40 hours.

Step #3: Calculating FTEs

Full-time equivalents (FTE) often suffer from mistaken identity. For instance, FTEs are thought to be people or jobs. In fact, FTEs are positions or hours worked. For example, two part-time RNs working half time will equate to 1 FTE, as their hours worked constitute the same as one full-time employee. One FTE equals 40 hours per week multiplied by 52 weeks, or 2,080 paid hours per year (some facilities use 2,096 hours to calculate paid hours per year—check with your finance department). Therefore, no matter how many part-time employees work, if their total hours worked equals 80 hours for that two-week pay period, then they equate to one FTE. (See Figure 4.3.)

FIGURE 4.3   **FTE calculation**

Hours worked per two-week period ÷ 80 hours = FTE			
RN Hours worked per two-week (80 hours) period			FTE
Sally	80	(80 ÷ 80 = 1.0)	1.0
Joe	72	(72 ÷ 80 = 0.9)	0.9
Steve	64	(64 ÷ 80 = 0.8)	0.8
Nancy	40	(40 ÷ 80 = 0.5)	0.5
Sam	24	(24 ÷ 80 = 0.2)	0.3
Betty	8	(8 ÷ 80 = 0.1)	0.1
How many employees are there?	6		
How many FTEs are there? **3.6 FTEs**			

Now it's time to calculate the number of productive FTEs budgeted for this year. To do this, use the following equation: total productive hours ÷ number of paid hours within a year for an FTE = total productive FTEs (67,500 ÷ 2,080 = 32.45 FTEs). This number helps you calculate future data. Based on your HPPD and UOS, your unit is budgeted for 32.45 total productive FTEs.

Calculating FTEs by staffs skill mix

According to Figure 4.2, the unit skill mix is 75% RN, 10% LVN, and 15% NA. Keeping that in mind, break down the FTEs further by their skill or job category. Do this by using the following equations:

- 75% (0.75) x 32.45 = 24.34 RN FTEs

- 10% (0.10) x 32.45 = 3.24 LPN FTEs

- 15% (0.15) x 32.45 = 4.87 NA FTEs
  Total = 32.45 FTEs

Step #4: Determining average hourly rate

The average hourly rate becomes more important when determining salaries for the year. By using the average hourly rate, you avoid having to use each staff member's hourly rate. However, for a more accurate calculation of salary expenses for next year, use each staff member's salary. Because this process is time-consuming, we will use the average hourly rate for the RN, LPN, and NA job categories in this book.

The average hourly rate can be obtained from numerous sources. Look at your recent labor distribution report, staffing offices computer-generated reports, or payroll department report. No matter how you obtain the average hourly rate, make sure you do, because it's necessary for determining total direct salaries. Be sure to get the average hourly rate for each job category.

Remember to factor in any projected merit increases/raises. To figure out the rate for each category, first determine the hours you will project for each productive category by using the following equations:

- RN total hours: 75% of 67,500 = 50,625 hours   (0.75 x 67,500 = 50,625)

- LPN total hours: 10% of 67,500 = 6,750 hours   (0.10 x 67,500 = 6,750)

- NA total hours: 15% of 67,500 = 10,125 hours   (0.15 x 67,500 = 10,125)

Step #5: Calculating salary dollars by skill mix

In Figure 4.4 you will find the hours worked by each skill category (i.e., RN, LPN, and NA), the categories average hourly pay rate, and the total direct salaries you must account for in the department's budget.

As you can see, by using the "average hourly rate" in the equation, you are able to get a more accurate projection for salaries than when using the unit average hourly rate.

FIGURE 4.4   **Sample total salaries calculation**

Hours x average hourly rate = Total direct salaries

RN: 50,625 x $25 = $1,265,625
LPN: 6,750 x $18 = $121,500
NA: 10,125 x $9 = $91,125
Total direct salary dollars =   **$1,478,250**

When using the unit average hourly rate, use following calculation:
67,500 x $17.33 = $1,169,775

Step #6: Determining replacement needs

Figuring replacement hours by skill category

Using the information found in Figure 4.4, the facility plans to spend approximately $1,478,250 for direct-care staff salaries for the year. However, when preparing your budget, remember that staff will take time off, and their replacement must be accounted for. To do this, first figure out the nonproductive hours, which will later be used to determine the cost of the replacement. The industry average for the percentage of nonproductive hours making up the total paid hours is 15%–20%. That means that 15%–20% of the money paid toward staff salaries is for nonproductive time (i.e., orientation, education, vacation, sick time, and holidays). This percentage varies depending on several factors such as the number of paid holidays the organization offers its employees as a benefit and orientation/education practices. The percentage of nonproductive hours is necessary when figuring FTEs and calculating the cost of salaries for the budget.

When budgeting for replacements, use 18% as the average (18% is the midpoint between 15%–20%, the industry average). This means that 18% of the time, the employee from this skill or job category will not be working. Therefore, replace 18% of that time and cost for each staff category. See Figure 4.5.

FIGURE 4.5   **Calculating replacement FTEs**

For varied skill mix
How many replacement FTEs do you need?
18% (0.18) x RN FTEs (24.34) = 4.4 FTEs
18% x LPN FTEs (3.24) = 0.58 FTEs
18% x NA FTEs (4.87) = 0.88 FTEs
Total additional FTEs needed for replacement: 5.86

For balanced skill mix
If staff skill mix is balanced at 50%/50% (i.e., 50% are RNs and 50% are LPNs), another way to calculate for replacement FTEs is by using the following equation:
Total FTEs x average replacement needed = Total additional FTEs needed for replacement
(32.45 x 0.18 = 5.84)

Now that you have figured out the additional FTEs needed for replacement staff, determine the new totals for the FTEs needed for next year.

- RN: 24.34 + 4.4 = 28.74

- LPN: 3.24 + 0.58 = 3.82

- NA: 4.87 + 0.88 = 5.75

- Total projected FTEs: 38.31

Now it's time to determine the amount of additional salaries that must be accounted for (nonproductive replacement) in the budget. See Figure 4.6.

FIGURE 4.6   **Determining nonproductive replacement**

How much additional salary do you need to pay for staff's allotted time off?
Total direct salaries x average replacement needed = Nonproductive replacement
($1,478,250 (see Figure 3.5) x 0.18 = $266,085)
Total additional salaries needed for replacement (nonproductive replacement) of 5.86 FTEs: $266,085

Let's calculate the amount of productive hours per FTE. See Figure 4.7.

FIGURE 4.7   Calculating productive hours per FTE

Adding cost of nonproductive replacement and additional FTEs to productive

Total direct salary dollars: $1,478,250	Total FTEs: 32.45 FTEs
Total nonproductive replacement: $266,085	Total nonprod. replacement: 5.86 FTEs
New total salaries: $1,744,335	**Total FTEs: 38.31 FTEs**

Because we are using 18% as an average for replacement, we know that 82% (100% –18% = 82%) of the total paid 2,080 hours per FTE are productive. This is figured by multiplying the total paid hours per FTE by the percent of productive hours (2,080 x 82%). Therefore, there are 1,706 productive hours per FTE. The remainder of the 2,080 hours per employee is used for vacations, holidays, sick time, etc.

Step #7: Determining expenses for indirect positions

For this example, assume the nurse manager and the monitor technician positions remain. Because the monitor technician is a 1.0 FTE on days, evenings, and nights and requires replacement, determine the total FTEs for this position by using the 18% replacement factor calculated earlier. For example, multiply the average replacement needed (18%) by monitor technician FTEs (3.0) to reach the nonproductive replacement (3.0 x 0.18 = 0.54). Then calculate the number of monitor technician FTEs by doing the following equation: 3.0 + 0.54 = 3.54 monitor technician FTEs. See Figure 4.8.

FIGURE 4.8   Sample position control

Position control			
	Approved	Filled	Status
Fixed staff			
Nurse manager	1.0		
Monitor technician	3.54		
Total fixed staff	**4.54**		
Variable staff			
RN (includes charge nurse)	28.73 (75% of 38.31)		
LPN	3.83 (10% of 38.31)		
NA	5.75 (15% of 38.31)		
Total variable staff	**38.31**		
Total positions	**42.85 FTEs**		

To update the position control, list currently filled positions and their status. This allows you to see which positions are open. See Figure 4.9.

FIGURE 4.9   **Updated position control**

Position control

	Approved	Filled	Status
Fixed staff			
Nurse manager	1.0	1.0	0
Monitor technician	3.54	3.25	0.29
Total fixed staff	4.54	4.25	0.29
Variable staff			
RN (includes charge nurse)	28.73	26.75 -	1.98
LPN	3.83	3.83	0
NA	5.75	6.0	+0.25
Total variable staff	38.31	36.58	1.73
Total positions:	**42.85**	**Total filled: 40.83**	**Total open: 2.02**

\+ FTEs are over the approved number
\- FTEs are under the approved number

You have calculated the direct salaries and replacements for the above salaries and FTEs. As you can see, other positions are considered indirect, as they do not provide hands-on patient care and are not part of the daily staffing hours. In this example, the nurse manager and monitor technician are considered indirect.

When adding the nurse manager and monitor technician's salaries, assume the nurse manager earns $75,000 per year and the technician makes $10 per hour. To figure out how much of the budget can be spent on the monitor technician's position, multiply the approved FTE (3.54) by the pay rate of the position. Then multiply that total by the number of hours per year (2,080; 3.54 x $10 x 2,080 = $73,632). Because the nurse manager is an FTE of 1.0 and is a salaried (or exempt) staff member, you do not have to multiply the salary amount by 2,080. To determine the total amount of indirect salary expenses that must be added to the current salary subtotal, add the two numbers together ($75,000 + $73,632 = $148,632). See Figure 4.10.

FIGURE 4.10 Determining total salaries

Total direct salaries:	$1,478,250	(See Figure 4.4)
Total nonproductive replacement:	$266,085	(See Figure 4.6)
Subtotal salaries:	$1,744,335	
Indirect staff salaries:	$148,632	(See calculation above)
Total salaries:	$1,892,967	

Step #8: Calculating skill mix of staff per shift

Now that you have figured out staff salaries, determine the skill mix of staff per shift. Remember that in some states, such as California, staffing ratios are mandated by law and dictate that nurses can only care for a specified number of residents at one time. It is likely that, in the future, other states will follow California's lead, so keep your ears and eyes open for changing legislation. For the purposes of the following exercise, assume that no such ratios exist. To determine skill mix, take factors such as your facility's policy, the level of resident acuity, resident care history, and staff competency, into consideration.

Your next action is to determine what percentage of nursing staff work days (7 a.m.–3 p.m.), evenings (3 p.m.–11 p.m.), and nights (11 p.m.–7 a.m.). Collaborate with staff when deciding the percentage of staff to work on each shift. For example, if the day shift is the busiest, consider putting most of your staff on the day shift. In units where activity does not change from shift to shift and shifts are generally eight hours long, (i.e., critical care), the allocation may be 33%/33%/33%. This is because work is evenly distributed among all shifts. Keep in mind that most activities occur during day and evening shifts.

For an active, 12-hour shift unit (i.e., in an intensive care unit), it may be 50%/50%. As nurse manager, you control this number and can make changes based on the unit's activity. However, you should involve your staff when deciding the best way to distribute work over the 24-hour period. Because each organization is different, there are no set standards for staff distribution except in areas mandated by regulations. For this example, use the information given in Figure 4.11. Also for this example, assume the following information is true:

- Budgeted ADC: 20.55
- HPPD: 9.0
- 75% of the staff are RNs
- 10% of the staff are LPNs
- 15% of the staff are NAs

FIGURE 4.11   Percentage of staff for each shift

Percentage of staff working days, evenings, and nights

1. Total direct-care hours ÷ number of days in a year = total hours of care per day
   67,500 ÷ 365 = 184.93 hours of care per day
2. Total hours of care per day ÷ length of shift = shifts for 24-hour period
   184.93 ÷ 8 hours shifts = 23.12 shifts
3. Ask staff to make a list of tasks and activities that occur routinely on each shift. This list should include medications, procedures, physician visits, orders, baths, ambulation, etc. The number of tasks per shift will determine the percentage of staff needed on each shift. For example, there are a total of 100 tasks: 40 performed on the day shift, 35 on the evening shift, and 25 on the night shift.

Staff distribution by shift: 40% days, 35% evenings, 25% nights

---

The amount of hours of care per day (184.93) helps you calculate the number of staff members needed to care for the ADC of 20.55 patients for seven days a week, 365 days a year. Remember FTEs are not shifts or people; they are positions or hours worked. To see what a 24-hour period would look like using the information calculated in Figure 4.11, review the chart in Figure 4.12. Using the following assumptions, you will be able to calculate how many shifts your department is allowed for a 24-hour period:

- Budgeted ADC: 20.55

- Total direct-care hours: 67,500

- Skill mix: 75% RN, 10% LPN, 15% NA

- Shift lengths: Eight hours

- Staff distribution by shift: 40% of X work days, 35% of X work evenings, 25% of X work nights

Use the following data to fill in the chart:

1. Total shifts for a 24-hour period

   - 67,500 ÷ 365 days = 184.93 hours per day ÷ eight-hour shifts = 23.12 shifts for a 24-hour period

2. Shifts per staff category for a 24-hour period

   - RN: 75% of 23.12 = 17.34 RN shifts for 24 hours

   - LPN: 10% of 23.12 = 2.31 LPN shifts for 24 hours

   - NA: 15% of 23.12 = 3.47 NA shifts for 24 hours

3. Number of staff needed to work shift (Finkler and Kovner 2000)

Days:

- 40% of the 17.34 RN shifts = 6.94

- 40% of the 2.31 LPN shifts = 0.92

- 40% of the 3.47 NA shifts = 1.39

Evenings:

- 35% of the 17.34 RN shifts = 6.07

- 35% of the 2.31 LPN shifts = 0.81

- 35% of the 3.47 NA shifts = 1.21

Nights:

- 25% of the 17.34 RN shifts = 4.34

- 25% of the 2.31 LPN shifts = 0.58

- 25% of the 3.47 NA shifts = 0.87

FIGURE 4.12 **Calculating the number of shifts needed per 24 hours**

Shift			Day (40%)	Evening (35%)	Night (25%)	Total
RN	(75%)	17.34	6.94	6.07	4.34	
LPN	(10%)	2.31	0.92	0.81	0.58	
NA	(15%)	3.47	1.39	1.21	0.87	
Total			**9.25**	**8.09**	**5.79**	**23.13**

After plotting the calculated numbers, you will notice figures such as 0.92 and 1.39. These figures represent the number of shifts that must be filled and the amount of RNs, LPNs, or NAs needed to do so. Decide whether to round such figures up or down. For instance, for the day shift, you are allowed to fill the schedule with 6.94 RNs, 0.92 LPNs, or 1.39 NAs. You decide whether to schedule six RNs, one LPN, and two NAs or seven RNs, one LPN, and one NA. Whatever you decide, be sure to base your decision on important factors such as your state's staffing regulations, department activity, and nurse competency.

FIGURE 4.13   **Number of shifts allowed per 24 hours**

Shift		Day (40%)	Evening (35%)	Night (25%)	Total
RN	(75%) 17.34	7	6	4	
LPN	(10%) 2.31	1	1	1	
NA	(15%) 3.47	1	1	1	
Total		9	8	6	23

Total number of shifts allowed per 24 hours: 23.13 shifts

Additional expenses

Additional salary expenses to add to the budget include shift differentials such as weekend bonuses, orientation, and benefits.

Step #9: Calculating differentials

Differentials are costs the facility pays to entice staff to work on the nonprime-time shifts such as evenings, nights, weekends, and holidays. Some facilities will even pay a differential to nurses willing to fill in as charge nurse. Differentials are used for those and other creative incentives to persuade staff to cover shifts they would not normally work. Every facility pays some form of differential, so it's important that you add these costs into your budget. Earlier, we calculated the average hourly rate, which was calculated on base hourly pay only. When calculating the average hourly rate for your unit, remember to include differentials in your math.

For the sake of this example, assume the facility pays the following differential:

Staff	Shift	Other
RN	3 p.m.–11 p.m.	$2.00
RN	11 p.m.–7 a.m.	$3.00
LPN	3 p.m.–11 p.m.	$1.50
LPN	11 p.m.–7 a.m.	$2.00
NA	3 p.m.–11 p.m.	$1.00
NA	11 p.m.–7 a.m.	$1.50

Remember that 40% of staff work the day shift, 35% work the evening shift, and 25% work the night shift. Use this information to calculate the additional salaries needed and add the sum to the salary subtotal. In other words, 40% of the staff will receive no differential because they are on the prime-time shift, 35% of the staff will receive the evening-shift differential, and 25% of the staff will receive the night-shift differential.

Determine the cost of such differentials by using the information we already have regarding skill mix and percentage of staff per shift. See Figures 4.14, 4.15, 4.16, and 4.17.

FIGURE 4.14   Calculating RN differential salary costs for evenings and nights

Total RN FTEs x percent that working shift = RN FTEs for the shift

Direct FTEs for RN: 75%
Total RN FTEs: 28.73
Work on evening shift: 35%   28.73 x 0.35 = 10.06 RN FTEs for the evening shift
Work on night shift: 25%   28.73 x 0.25 = 7.18 RN FTEs for the night shift
Average hourly rate (See Figure 3.3 on page 48): $25/hour

RN FTE for the shift x differential expense x number of hours per year = differential salary expenses for RNs
Evening shift: 10.06 x $2 x 2,080 = **$41,850**
Night shift: 7.18 x $3 x 2,080 = **$44,803**

FIGURE 4.15   Calculating LPN differential salary costs for evenings and nights

Total LPN x percent that working shift = LPN FTEs for the shift

Direct FTEs for LPN: 10%
Total LPN FTEs: 3.82
Work on evening shift: 35%   3.82 x 0.35 = 1.34 LPN FTEs for the evening shift
Work on night shift: 25%   3.82 x 0.25 = 0.96 LPN FTEs for the night shift
Average hourly rate: $18/hour

LPN for the shift x differential expense x number of hours per year = differential salary expenses for LPNs
Evening shift: 1.34 x $1.50 x 2,080 = **$4,181**
Night shift: 0.96 x $2 x 2,080 = **$3,994**

FIGURE 4.16   Calculating FTEs differential salary costs for evenings and nights

Total NA FTEs x percent that working shift = NA FTEs for the shift

Direct FTEs for NA: 15%
Total NA FTEs: 5.75
Work on evening shift: 35%   5.75 x 0.35 = 2.01 NA FTEs for the evening shift
Work on night shift: 25%   5.75 x 0.25 = 1.43 NA FTEs for the night shift
Average hourly rate: $9/hour

NA FTE for the shift x differential expense x number of hours per year = Differential salary expenses for NAs
Evening shift: 2.01 x $1 x 2,080 = **$4,180**
Night shift: 1.43 x $1.50 x 2,080 = **$4,462**

FIGURE 4.17   Total shift differentials

	Evening shift	Night shift
RN	$41,850	$44,803
LPN	4,181	3,994
NA	4,180	4,462
Total	50,211 +	53,259 = $103,470

Step #10: Totaling salaries
Now that you've calculated shift differentials, retally the total for salaries and the budget.
(See Step #6.)

Total direct salaries:	$1,478,250
Total nonproductive replacement:	266,085
Subtotal salaries:	$1,744,335
Indirect staff salaries from above:	148,632
Total salaries:	$1,892,967
Shift differentials:	103,470
New total:	$1,996,437

If you work in a facility that pays additional differentials to nurses filling in as charge nurse, remember to add the additional expenses to the final total. Use the following formula to calculate the additional salary cost:

Average number of nurses filling in as charge nurse x number of hours per week x 52 weeks x differential ($1/hour) = Total amount for charge nurse differential (10 nurses x 8 hours x 52 x $1 = $4,160)

Step #11: Figuring benefits

Benefits, or fringe benefits, are the last wages calculated and added to this section of expenses. Benefits are special perks given to those employed by the facility. Such benefits may include medical, dental, vision, and life insurance. They also include pension and Social Security.

Today, benefits constitute 25%–35% of salary expenses. Check with the finance department for your facility's benefits percentage. For this example, use the benefits percentage of 30%. Add benefits to the total direct and indirect salary expense. To figure the amount of the budget spent on benefits, multiply the total salary expense by the percentage of benefits ($1,996,437 x 30% = $598,931).

Step #12: Calculating overtime

Pay close attention to incremental overtime. For instance, if staff routinely stay late to complete patient charts, talk, etc., their extra overtime minutes can add up.

If your facility allows you to budget for overtime—some facilities do not—review the previous year's data and calculate overtime at the facility's overtime rate of pay. For example, if the overtime rate is time and a half and an RN makes $25/hour, the overtime rate of pay is $37.50/hour. To figure out how much overtime the RN would make, multiply the overtime rate of pay by the number of hours of overtime projected and the total added to the salaries. For example, assume each RN works an average of 10 overtime hours per year. Use the following formula to calculate the cost of overtime:

Average overtime hours per year (10 hours) x overtime rate ($37.50) x the RN FTE (28.73) = Total cost of RN overtime (10 x $37.50 x 28.73 = $10,774).

Scheduled overtime is the overtime that is planned for in your budget. It can be the last four hours of a 12-hour shift or planned extra shifts. Some facilities are strict about overtime and only allow scheduled or 12-hour shift overtime be budgeted with the understanding that the manager will control it. In such cases, overtime is not allowed unless it is an emergency. However, this practice is facility-specific, so ask about your organization's policy. For this book, assume that no overtime has been budgeted for the coming year.

Step #13: Determining orientation and education/training costs

Orientation is the period of time set aside for new hires to learn policies and procedures and to become acclimated with its activities. Orientation consists of reading policies, observing experienced nurses, performing return demonstrations of tasks, caring for residents under supervision, and gaining understanding of unit practice standards.

When budgeting for orientation, either set money aside to pay for it or combine it with education. In some cases, orientation even may fall under productive hours. (It is important to understand where these orientation dollars are located so you can budget accordingly.) For instance, if you expect to absorb the orientation costs into productive HPPD, then factor this into your schedule. In other words, leave a buffer for those days when you have orientees on the unit.

Critical thinking

For this activity, assume that education, training, and orientation are separate from the HPPD and have a line item to themselves.

Facts:

- You will hire five new RNs and one LPN this year

- Each new RN and LPN requires six weeks of orientation on the day shift

- You will hire two new NAs this year

- Each new NA requires four weeks of orientation on the day shift

- Everyone on the staff is entitled to five paid education days per year

- All staff are paid to attend six two-hour-long staff meetings

- All staff are paid to attend four hours of cardiopulmonary resuscitation (CPR) training

- All RNs must take an eight-hour advanced cardiac life support (ACLS) course every two years

See Figures 4.18, 4.19, and 4.20.

FIGURE 4.18 **Calculating orientation costs for new hires**

> **Number of hires X length of orientation (in hours) X average hourly rate = total orientation costs**
>
> RN: 5 x 6 weeks (240 hours) x $25 = $ 30,000
> LPN: 1 x 6 weeks (240 hours) x $18 = $4,320
> NA: 2 x 4 weeks (160 hours) x $9 = $2,880
> Total hours: 640 (total hours) ÷ by 2,080 = additional 0.3 FTE of staff for orientation. This number (0.3) must be added to the total budgeted FTEs.

FIGURE 4.19   Calculating education and training costs for new hires

---

FTE x paid education hours + (CPR training hours + staff meeting hours) = Total education and training hours A
5 days = 40 hours, 4 hours + 12 hours = 16 hours, 40 + 12 = 56 hours
RN: 28.74 x 56 hours = 1,609 hours
Because the eight-hour ACLS is required every two years, you will budget 50% for the first year and 50% for the second. Therefore, only 50% of RNs will take the course this year.

50% of RNs x hours of ACLS training = Total education and training hours B
50% of RNs (14.37) x 8 = 114.96, or 115 hours
(Total education and training hours A + total education and training hours B) x average hourly rate = total education and training costs
(1,609 + 115) x $25 = $43,100

FTE x paid education hours + (CPR training hours + staff meeting hours) x average hourly rate = total education and training hours
LPN: 3.82 x 56 hours x $18 = $3,851
NA: 5.75 x 56 hours x $9 = $2,898

FIGURE 4.20   Calculating total orientation and education/
                    training costs for new hires

Total orientation costs + total education/training costs = total orientation and education/training costs

RN: $30,000 + 43,100 = $73,100
LPN: $4,320 + $3,851 = $8,171
NA: $2,880 + $2,898 = $5,778

Total orientation and education/training costs for RN + total for LPN + total for NA = total orientation and education/training costs
$73,100 + $8,171 + $5,778 = $87,049
You must add $87,049 orientation and education/training costs to the 2005 budget.

Now, total up the salaries for the budget:

Total direct salaries:	$1,478,250
Total nonproductive replacement:	266,085
Subtotal salaries:	$1,744,335
Indirect staff salaries from above:	148,632
Subtotal salaries:	$1,892,967
Shift differentials:	103,470
Benefits:	598,931
Subtotal salaries:	$2,595,368
Orientation:	87,049
Grand total salaries:	$2,682,417

Variable costs vs. fixed costs

For budgeting purposes, all costs are considered to be either fixed or variable. A variable cost is a cost or expense that is incurred as a direct result of volume (i.e., increased census). A fixed cost is one the unit will experience regardless of the volume or activity (i.e., the electricity bill). The following are examples of both:

Variable costs	Fixed costs
Personnel	Electricity
Education	Depreciation
Food	Preventative maintenance
Supplies	Xerox rental
Linen	Nurse manager salary

Variable costs are budgeted based on the UOS. That is because supply use increases and decreases with patient census. Fixed costs, on the other hand, are often divided and budgeted as a flat monthly rate.

When budgeting for nonsalary items such as supplies, the finance department should provide you with an "inflation factor." (If they do not, however, you must do the necessary research to obtain the number.) The inflation factor is a predetermined number accounting for price increases for the coming year. For the purposes of this chapter, assume the inflation factor is 6%.

Annualizing costs

One of the most common methods for annualizing costs is to look at the year-to-date (YTD) data on the most current departmental reports. "Annualizing" allows you to estimate the end-of-the-year, or YTD, numbers based on the unit's monthly history. Assuming there is data for the past eight months, to project expenses for the upcoming year, divide the YTD total—which is found on the departmental financial statement/cost-center report—by eight to get an average monthly expense. Then, multiply the sum by 12 months to reach an annualized number.

For example, the YTD expenses for supplies is $35,000.

YTD expense ÷ number of months of data = average monthly expense x number of months in a year = annualized expense ($35,000 ÷ 8 = $4,375 x 12 = $52,500)

Although this method is not always exact, it does give you an estimate for average monthly expenses. After calculating the average for eight months of data, try to think of any significant expenses that may be incurred for the next four months that would be reflected in the average. If any, add them into the total. For example, if the average monthly expense is $4,375 and next month you expect to add a large volume of a new supply item to the supply cart, add this amount to the supply budget total. (See Figure 4.21.)

FIGURE 4.21 **Methods for annualizing costs and planning expenses**

> **Methods for annualizing costs and planning next year's expenses**
>
> **Total fixed cost expenses YTD x 8 months x 12 months = Annualized figure**
>
> Fixed costs:
> Bio-med costs for the last 8 months = $2,500.
> ($2,500 ÷ 8) x 12 months = $3,750 annualized figure
> For next year's budget:
>
> **Annualized figure x inflation factor = Expenses for next year's budget**
> $3,750 x 6% (1.06) = $3,975 for next year's budget

Supplies

To determine supply expenses for the unit, review Figure 4.22.

FIGURE 4.22 **Supply budgeting**

> For the first eight months of this year, your unit consumed the following in supplies:
>
> Medical = $23,967
> $23,967 ÷ 8 x 12 = $35,951 x 1.06 = **$38,108 projected for next year**
>
> Nonmedical = $12,006
> $12,006 ÷ 8 x 12 = $18,009 x 1.06 = **$19,090 projected for next year**

Plugging in your budget numbers

Now it's time to plot the above figures into your budget. See the example for the medical-surgical/telemetry unit in Figure 4.23.

FIGURE 4.23   **2009 budget**

Budget for 2009	
Patient days	**7,500**
Revenue	**5,950,000**
Expenses	
Direct salaries	$1,478,250
Nonproductive salaries	266,085
Indirect salaries	148,632
Differentials/bonuses	103,470
Orientation/training	87,049
Overtime	0
Employee benefits	598,931
Total salaries	**$2,682,417**
Medical supplies	38,108
Nonmedical supplies	19,090
Minor equipment	1,800
Equipment rental	807
Maintenance	1,506
Bio-med	3,975
Linen	14,080
Nutritional support	20,948
Interdepartmental transfers	23,889
Other	1,109
Total other expenses	**125,312**
Total expenses	**$2,807,729**

Capital budgets

A capital budget is one that outlines projected buying of large, fixed assets or equipment that depreciates such as MRI or ultrasound machines. What qualifies as a capital expense varies among organizations; however, generally, it is any piece of equipment that is worth more than $500 and has a lifespan of five years.

The capital budget is separate from the operating budget and requires all requests for capital equipment be approved by a budget committee. Granted requests must meet the goals and objectives of the hospital.

If you are responsible for developing a capital budget, you may have to fill out a form called the "capital budget acquisition form." Such forms are used when requesting funding for new equipment. They are used to make the case for purchasing new, large price-tag items and equipment.

Position control

The position control, or position budget (approved positions), discussed in step #7, is an important document and resource, second only to the budget itself. The position control identifies each job category, the number of budgeted FTEs, and whether projections are on target or there are vacant positions. The position control also indicates whether there are too many positions for a particular job category.

The position control comes in several varieties, and it was long thought that its only purpose was to serve as the "hiring plan" for the unit and for human resources (HR). However, when it is used as the translation of the budget into the defined "scheduling requirements" for the unit, it takes on greater importance in providing staffing for safe patient outcomes because there is consistent evidence for an association between the level of nursing staffing and resident outcomes.

Be sure to update the position control regularly as it changes each budget year or as your number of FTEs and skill mix change. In fact, update the position control each time a person is hired or when an employee resigns, transfers, or changes status.

Minimum, good, and best position control management

According to the Labor Management Institute, at a minimum, position control management addresses filled and open positions compared to hired and actual FTE positions.

Good position control addresses the minimum requirements as well as:

Incorporates or references the budgeted FTEs by skill mix

- Positions by job codes or classes or skill mix (e.g., RN, LPN, NA) for direct care (defined as those that are part of the variable staffing plan providing hands-on care to the patient)

- Positions by job codes or classes or skill mix for indirect care (defined as those that are paid from the cost center but are not part of the variable staffing plan [also called fixed staff])

- – The "best" position control will include:

  - – Job codes to track budgeted dollars for your FTE positions

  - – Hire dates for the employees in the filled positions to track issues regarding seniority

  - – Designation for full-time (FT) or part-time (PT) status as a check for your optimum or budgeted FT/PT rotation plan

- Position control numbering schemas that allow for "loaning" filled positions to other units for some period (e.g., a diabetic educator that is hired to a unit for a diabetic education program that gets put on hold)

- Position control reports that provide:

  - – Tracking by shift as a check against your budgeted "care distribution hours"

- Position tracking for weekday and weekend distribution to:

  - – Compare your budgeted positions to the schedule at posting to visually check that you have distributed your resources to the shifts to which they

  - – are budgeted

  - – Compare your budgeted positions to the schedule after the schedule is posted to visually establish where your resources ended up working, especially if you use self-scheduling in your unit (or selfish scheduling, depending on your unit-based guidelines and employee requests)

- Comparison of actual to budget paid FTEs with variance

- Comparison of actual worked FTEs to the target or variable staffing plan FTEs with variance

- Comparison of actual and budget workload for productivity reference (e.g., how busy the unit was for the period being evaluated)

Please refer to the position control example shown in Figure 4.24, which is the summary portion of the position control plan that demonstrates, integrates, and compares the unit's budget to the position control plan. It also contains the budgeted-job codes, the position control numbers (e.g., 902.691.1201.1966.1) that incorporate the unit's cost center (902), the job code (e.g., 691), and the employee's hire date.

FIGURE 4.24 Position Control Example

	Total	700	1500	2300	Nonproductive data		Per day	0700 Pos. Hours	1500 Pos. Hours	2300 Pos. Hours
Unit Budget FTEs	43.7	14.6	14.6	14.6	Budget NP%	9.70%				
Position control FTEs	43.7	14.6	14.6	14.6	Budget NP hours	8,819.20	24	8	8	8
Hired FTEs	40.8				Budget NP FTEs	4.24				
Direct HPPD	19.5	6.5	6.5	6.5	Unit replacement NP FTE allocation	2.24	12.73			
Total HPPD	22.7	7.6	7.6	7.6	Resource Pool NP FTE Allocation	2	12			

Job Code	Job Title	Position Number	PC FTE	Hired FTE	Var. FTE	Filed By	Hire Date	Status	0700 Pos. Hours	1500 Pos. Hours	2300 Pos. Hours
691		902.691.12011996.1	0.9	0.9	0	PT	12-01-1996	FT		32	40
692		902.692.12121999.1	0.9	0.9	0	JC	12-12-1999	FT		32	40
		Filled RN Positions	31.8	31.8	0.05				9.35	12.15	10.3
		902.682.00000000.1	1	0	-1	Vacant					80
		902.682.00000000.2	1	0	-1	Vacant					80
		902.682.00000000.3	0.2	0	-0.2	Vacant					16
		Vacant RN Positions	2.2	0	2.3				0	0	2.2
		Total RN's=34.1	34.1	31.8	2.3				9.35	12.15	12.6
		Total RNs	34.1	31.8	2.3						
		Total Care Partners	3	2.5	0.6						
		Total Direct	37.1	34.2	2.9						
		Total Indirect	6.6	6.6	0						
		Total FTEs	43.7	40.8	2.9				14.55	14.55	14.6

RN Weekend Program

Overtime in excess of 5% is associated with adverse patient outcomes (medication errors and patient falls) based on research conducted by the Labor Management Institute, so position control reports that can tell us how efficiently and effectively we are scheduling and staffing our resources should help us to promote safe staffing for our patients. I recommend the *Position Control Best Practice Guidelines* developed by the Labor Management Institute. See Figure 4.25 for the Labor Management Institute's criteria to help you evaluate your position control.

FIGURE 4.25   Labor Management Institute best practices position control

| Name: _____ | Unit name: _____ |

Instructions: As a manager, please indicate if you are provided the criteria necessary to evaluate your position control comments. Thank you.

Criteria for evaluation of cost center position control:	Responses	
	Yes	No
1. Based on the budgeted FTE's		
2. Includes filled and unfilled (vacant FTE's)		
3. Includes category of staff (job codes/classes) or skill mix (for example, caregiver groups such as direct: RN, LPN, NA, other and indirect: e.g., unit manager, secretary)		
4. Includes date of hire for seniority tracking		
5. Includes positions for both full-time and part-time work agreements		
6. Allows positions to be distributed by shifts (days, p.m., and nights)		
7. Allows positions to be distributed on weekends		
8. Compares budgeted positions to filled positions		
9. Compares actual hours worked by shift to the budgeted position		
10. Compares overtime by shift to the budgeted position		
11. Compares agency/traveler hours by shift to the budgeted positions		
12. Compares actual and budgted census or other workload for the reporting period		
13. Is managed by the unit manager		
14. Is shared by HR as the unit's hiring plan		
15. Is shared by finance for FTE management		
16. Is integrated to and updated automatically by HR, payroll, and workload information		
17. Provides reports that have been updated from integrated system data		

Source: 2002-2007 © Labor Management Institute and ChrysMarie Suby. Used with permission.

Once you determine the number of FTEs needed for the budget, develop a list of positions broken down by category. See Figure 4.8 for a sample position control.

Interviewing and hiring

Despite the many refinements that have been developed in recruiting and screening methods, the interview is still considered the most vital part of the selection process. The interview offers both the prospective employee and the employer the opportunity to obtain information, gather impressions, and make observations that would not be possible otherwise.

Normally, the objectives of the selection interview are to:

- Allow the interviewer to obtain the required knowledge about the applicant to determine whether he or she is suitable for employment in a particular position

- Provide sufficient information about the organization and the particular job so the applicant can make a decision of acceptance or rejection

- Treat the applicant in a manner that will create and maintain goodwill toward the organization

Review the job description

It is critical to have an up-to-date job description that provides clear job requirements for both the hiring manager and the prospective employee.

Make sure the job description accurately and realistically reflects the essential duties and requirements of the job. Think about the skills, knowledge, and abilities needed to perform it successfully.

A job description helps to.

- Give applicants an accurate description of the job and its requirements

- Focus your attention on key language for job advertisements and interview questions that are critical in recruiting top talent

- Provide you and the employee with a foundation on which to base performance and future growth

Finding the "right fit"

The ultimate goal of interviewing and selecting staff is to find the right fit between the talents, skills, and abilities needed in a given role and the talents, skills, and abilities of a given applicant. Remember to "hire for talent, knowing that you can train for skills." Using this approach requires that some thought be given to the process:

- Review the job description to consider the talents needed in the role, such as a "take-charge style" or "attention to detail" or being "self-directed"

- Study your best staff to determine the talents they bring to their roles, such as the ability to manage multiple priorities or mentorship of others

- Identify one or two critical talents that can be the focus during the interview

- Consider both the current and future needs of the unit, such as an upcoming computer installation or an organizational initiative on customer service, so that these can be addressed during the interview

Face-to-face interviews

The purpose of the face-to-face interview is to further narrow your initial group of applicants by learning as much about them as possible in a relatively limited time. This is a fact-finding mission for both parties, as both need information to ensure a successful outcome.

Interview questions

Asking the right questions in interviews can help managers get answers that will enable them to select the right candidate for the right job.

Some applicants are very rehearsed. They know how to anticipate or deflect difficult questions. They know the "correct" answer to many questions, mainly because they have been asked the same questions over and over or have a written script that anticipates questions. To limit canned answers, formulate questions that cannot be anticipated by the applicant. These questions should be original and are less commonly asked by interviewers, and they will lessen the possibility of evoking canned responses.

Past behavior is the best indication you will have of future behavior. As you seek to find a good fit in the interviewing process, "tell me about a time when" questions will serve you well.

Question types

1. Behavioral interview questions.

Behavioral interviewing techniques probe beyond superficial answers, requiring candidates to assess themselves and recall examples of behavior. Most behavioral questions are formed as either self-appraisal queries or situational queries, as shown in the examples below:

Self-appraisal queries:

- "If you had the choice between working in a job with peaks and valleys in the workload or working in a job with a steady volume of work, which would you choose and why?"

- "What have you learned from mistakes you have made in the past?"

- "If I were to call the references you have listed, what would they say about you?"

Situational query:

- "Tell me about a time when you had to make a critical decision in your manager's absence. How did you handle it?"

- "When was the last time you had to break or bend the rules, and how did you do it?"

2. Open-ended questions.

These questions require an explanation from the candidate. Open-ended questions begin with words such as, "what," "why," "how," "describe," and "explain." For example:

- "What is the greatest asset you will bring to this job?"

- "What about this job comes naturally to you?"

- "Tell me about the last time you had a short deadline and how you handled it."

- "How have you had to adapt to your job's changing needs?"

- "What approach to solving work-related problems seems to work best for you?"

3. Neutral questions.

Neutral questions do not reveal a bias toward an acceptable or correct answer. For example, "If you had to choose between one extreme or the other, would you want a supervisor who leaves you alone to get your work done and only wants to hear from you if there's a problem, or would you prefer someone who meets with you regularly to help you focus on your goals for the day or week?"

4. Yes or no questions.

Use questions that can be answered with a "yes" or "no" to confirm information you already have. In general, use these types of questions sparingly because they do not add new information. For example, "Were you with XYZ company for 10 years before you relocated to San Francisco?"

5. Follow-up questions.

After a candidate answers a question, follow up with another question that probes the candidate's attitudes or delves further into the issue. For example, you may start with a broad question such as, "What are your responsibilities as the administrative assistant?" A candidate may respond with a list of duties, such as answering phones, typing, keeping the calendar, arranging travel, and filing documents. Although this information confirms the resume, it does not give information about the relationship with the supervisor, consequences of actions, or pride in work output. To get this kind of information, ask follow-up questions, such as:

- "What aspects of your job are most satisfying?"

- "What kinds of things do you learn easily?"

- "What skills do you need to improve in the next year?"

- "What about your previous employment did you find the most frustrating?"

- "What did you most appreciate about the managers you have had in the past?"

- "In reflecting on your professional experience, of what are you most proud?"

- "Where do you see yourself five years from now?"

- "In relating to others, do you consider yourself an introvert or an extrovert?"

Remember that interview questions must focus on job-related areas only, without any reference to race, sex, age, religion, national origin, marital status, sexual orientation, or apparent or perceived mental or physical disabilities. They must focus on the applicant's ability to do the job.

Questions not to ask

Avoid unintentionally discriminatory questions that violate equal opportunity laws, including but not limited to the following:

- "What year did you graduate from high school?"

- "Where were you born?"

- "Where did you learn a foreign language?"

- "What are your child-care arrangements?"

- "What are your religious practices?"

- "How many days did you miss because of illness last year?

- "Do you have any disabilities?"

- "Have you ever been arrested?"

Tips for a successful interview

The environment

It helps to give some thought ahead of time to the physical environment in which you will conduct the interview. You will want to find a private area in which you can spend enough uninterrupted time. Applicants will be more at ease and you will learn more about them in an environment that is not threatening.

Preparing yourself

Discuss with a representative in the HR department the information obtained on the application, including references, and whether they will make the salary quote or have you conduct that aspect of the interview. If you will be sharing a salary range with the applicant, verify your information with HR for accuracy. Review the information on the applicant just before the interview so that the details are fresh in your mind. Be sure to look for and possibly ask about on the interview:

- **Gaps in employment**
  Do not assume they were caused by negative reasons.

- **Special skills**
  Are they experts with certain computer software? Ask for examples of these skills.

- **Level of responsibility**

  When applicants use words such as "assisted" and "arranged" when describing a project, they often mean that they were involved in a project but not actually responsible for it. Explore
  this further.

- **Job longevity**

  This can be a good sign of a person's loyalty to his or her employer.

- **Many short-term jobs**

  This can be a sign that the person is not loyal to his or her employer. You should ask in detail why the applicant made each move from job to job to understand the motivation behind it.

Preparing the applicant

Just as it is important to prepare yourself for the interview, preparing the applicant can save you time during the interview and help make your decision. If the interview is scheduled, mail the perspective candidate a letter verifying the date, time, and location and mention that you look forward to meeting him or her. Include a copy of the mission statement and the job description, and ask the applicant to review them in preparation for the interview. At the time of your meeting, begin with some questions related to the letter and its contents. If the applicant obviously did not review them to prepare for the interview, no matter how "qualified" he or she may seem, this behavior will not change. If the mission statement and job description were not important enough to read in preparation for the interview, they will not become any more important to the applicant if you hire him or her.

Conducting the interview

There is no specific recipe for conducting a good interview that will work for all applicants, so you will have to adapt your style to each applicant you meet. For example, there are shy people who appreciate it when the interviewer makes them comfortable with a little small talk in the beginning of the interview. You may want to start by commenting on a neutral subject (e.g., the weather) to break the ice a bit. Then, you can let the applicant know who you are relative to the position. Are you the immediate supervisor? Will you be making the hiring decision? Will you discuss the pay and benefits with them, or will they be talking to someone else about these issues?

Note taking

Even though you may think that you will remember everything about an applicant you have interviewed, most of us do not. Notes are helpful when several top applicants emerge and close comparison becomes necessary. Mention to the applicant that you will be taking notes—doing so up front makes him or her feel more comfortable. Limit note taking to short entries—it is more important to listen—and allow time to go over the notes immediately after the interview. Refine the notes by writing a summary of each interviewed applicant for later comparison. Do not write your notes on the resume/application. Take notes on a separate piece of paper.

Establish a friendly tone, but manage the interview

Make certain that you control the interview; don't let forceful applicants talk incessantly or take the lead. Use the interview time efficiently to get your most important questions answered.

Make the interview accessible to people with disabilities

But don't question the nature, severity, cause, or expected outcome of disabilities. Focus on the essential functions and attendance standards of the job. Do not make assumptions based on actual or perceived disabilities. Ask all applicants the same questions regardless of whether they have actual or perceived disabilities.

Have the applicant do most of the talking

Apply the 70/30 rule: The applicant talks 70% of the time; you talk 30% of the time. You will want to provide some general information about your department, philosophy, and culture, but keep your comments brief. The main purpose of the interview is to gather as much information as possible from the applicant.

Allow silence

During the interview, the applicant needs time to think. If an applicant seems reluctant to answer a difficult question, don't rush on to the next question to make the applicant feel more comfortable. An awkward silence can indicate that you have reached an area you may want to probe further, or it could simply mean the applicant cannot think of an immediate answer.

If applicants falsely represent their qualifications . . .

End the interview early, although you should try to do so in a neutral rather than accusatory way. If, on the other hand, it becomes clear that you simply misunderstood the applicant's qualifications and they are not a fit with the job's requirements, show them the courtesy of completing the interview, although you will probably want to shorten it somewhat.

Handling awkward responses

Applicants sometimes volunteer information that employers may not lawfully consider when evaluating an applicant for a position. For example, they may tell you, "I have two children."

"We are expecting a baby." "My spouse is disabled." Do not follow up on this information even though the applicant brought it to your attention. The best way to handle this situation is to acknowledge what was said simply by nodding and saying, "Oh," "I see," or another similarly neutral comment. Then continue with your next prepared question related to the position.

Hasty judgments

Many interviewers find themselves making up their minds about applicants very early on in the interview—sometimes as early as the minute the person walks in the door. This rush to judgment can be very detrimental to a well-thought-out hiring process. Once you sense that you are forming an opinion about the applicant, either positive or negative, ask questions specifically to find out if your impression is correct. You may confirm what you have already sensed, or you may be surprised to discover that the applicant has characteristics or traits that you completely missed in your initial assessment.

Tell the applicant about the job and about working for your organization

Be sure to allow enough time to talk in more detail about the job opening, provide an overview of your department's structure, how it fits into the institution as a whole, etc. You should also allow some time for applicants to ask you more questions based on what you say. Pay attention to the kinds of questions they ask: they can tell you a lot about their interest level in the job. Share the mission statement with them, and ask them for an example of how they could apply it in the patient care area.

Allow some time for applicants to ask you more questions

They will have questions about the organization, benefits, why you came to work there, or your style of management. You should be prepared to answer, although briefly, questions about yourself, background or history of the unit, the work culture, characteristics of the physician staff, and other questions particular to the job opening. You should also be prepared to sell the job to a good applicant and show how attractive it would be to work at your facility if the offer were ultimately made. However, never mislead even the best of candidates to encourage them to take the position. Always be honest in your responses. If they ask you about recent financial challenges, layoffs, etc., respond candidly and then follow up with something positive such as, "Did you notice that we offer onsite dry cleaning drop off/pick up, child care, and Wednesday take-home suppers from our cafeteria?"

The peer-interviewing process

Having completed your interview of the applicant, explain how staff will be taking part in the process. It is important that the applicant understand that you routinely involve the staff it interviewing applicants and that, although you will be making the final decision, the input from staff will have considerable weight in determining which candidate is a good fit for the unit. Also, because staff have first-hand experience of what the job requires, they are in a good position to give the applicant information that could be helpful.

Make the applicant aware that their resume will be shared with the staff involved in the interview process. Give the applicant an expected time frame for the peer interview and background information about the interview team. Also share with the applicant the process by which they will be contacted for the peer interview as well as a time frame in which you plan to make your final decision.

Peer interviewing

Although the process of developing a peer interview team may take time and preparation, studies have shown that peer interviews increase the likelihood that staff will be welcoming and supportive of new hires and that they improve fit and compatibility. In a staff meeting, solicit feedback as to who staff would like to have as their interview team (usually including three to five team members).

You will need to have at least one or two coaching sessions with this team so that they feel prepared and confident in the interview process. This coaching should include the tips in this section that you have found helpful, and the following do's and don'ts:

Do
- Know the questions you can and cannot ask in the interview
- Apply the 70/30 rule
- Believe the answer you get, not what you would like to hear
- Use behavioral interview questions
- Listen for talents (i.e., what do they learn easily or what comes naturally to them) rather than solely skills and experience

Don't

- Contrast applicants with one with another

- Be influenced by first impressions

- Fall victim to the "halo" effect (i.e, finding an applicant very likable or charismatic and ignoring other information that would indicate the lack of a good fit for the role)

Interview teams often find it helpful to discuss the talents needed in the role and to focus on one or two they consider crucial as well as making a list of the key technical skills and interpersonal skills needed in the role. Listing these in a chart format for use in note taking during each interview allows for more consistency in the interviews and assists the interview team in formulating their recommendation.

Evaluation

Once you have the team's input, you will need to evaluate it and take into consideration that different people react differently to the same applicant, even to the same answers. Listen to your interview team members to understand their reasoning and ask questions if your interview with the same applicant left a significantly different impression. You will need to use your best judgment, but factoring in the feedback from the peer interviews is vital. If you find that your selection differs from the interview team's, then explain the reasons for your decision to the team and make every effort to reach a decision you can all support. Remember that the interview team will be more invested in the process if they see that their decisions are heavily weighted in the process.

Make the offer and close out the process

You have made your choice and are ready to make the offer. Contact your HR at this stage, as they can assist you in determining the appropriate hiring salary and completing the necessary documentation on recruitment for the job.

It is a both polite and good business practice to notify the remaining applicants that your offer was accepted by another applicant. It sends a message to applicants that your company is professional and respectful in how it conducts business and appreciates that candidates have taken the time to apply. In addition, the second or third choice applicant could very well be the next hire when another job becomes available, so it's important to end the process on a professional, friendly note.

A short note or telephone call informing applicants of the decision is appropriate. If you choose to make a phone call, keep in mind that they can be difficult because the applicant may ask why he or she was not chosen. It is best to keep these conversations short and not to get into any kind of debate. The reason for not hiring someone can always be stated simply: You found an applicant whose skills and abilities you think will best fit the position.

When you present a problem or concern to me I will expect you to put it in writing with your name and your recommendations of at least two reasonable resolutions to the situation/problem. Why am I doing this? Because you are the ones out in the patient-care area, and you know what works well with the systems we have in place. Secondly, your job descriptions require each of you to participate in the problem-solving process, so if you identify a problem, you should be accountable and willing to help fix it. Does anyone have any questions?

How will staff react? Picture yourself surrounded by several unhappy campers, alongside some individuals who are saying to themselves, "Well, it's about time!"

To help this process become effective for staff, you should consider holding a meeting where staff decide, as a team, what the acceptable and unacceptable behaviors will be for the department. Ask staff to write on index cards two behaviors they believe to be unacceptable for members of the department. Start them off with examples such as "the use of foul language" or "speaking negatively about another staff member in front of patient/family." Then have a staff member collect all of the cards and read them to another staff member, who should write them on a flip chart or white board. Identify the items most often noted by staff—they become the beginning of their accountabilities. Have them typed up, require all staff to sign them, and post them so they are visible to staff. At each staff meeting, determine whether there are any new items staff want added to the list (and there will be). Keep the list updated with new signatures, and once the list is finalized, revisit it once a year.

This process places the responsibilities directly on the peer group and takes them off the manager. They have determined what is unacceptable. Therefore, when they start complaining or whining about one another and they are unwilling to help resolve the problem, pull out the sheet with their signature and their job description (with statement about actively participating in problem solving) and address the issue from those perspectives.

However, be careful that you do not completely pull yourself out of the resolution loop. As manager, you are still responsible for overseeing their actions and approving their recommendations, when appropriate. If, for example, a staff member feels someone they work with isn't carrying their share of the work load, it is still your responsibility to determine whether you need to step in and reclarify job descriptions or to determine whether there is a personality conflict interfering with patient care.

"How much grief could be avoided if everyone at the workplace simply practiced a bit of consideration and courtesy?" —Andrew S. Grove, CEO, Intel Corp.

What do I do when a staff member raises a grievance with me?

To a staff grievance, you should always respond seriously to a staff grievance, and in a manner that respects the confidentiality of all parties. You should endeavor to resolve it promptly, with a minimum of stress to all parties, and follow the principles of procedural fairness.

Gathering facts on grievances is essential to the proper consideration of and response to them. Before considering any grievance, it is imperative to ensure that all the facts of the case have been collected. Never fail to interview the grievor to get his or her viewpoint.

Effectively resolving conflict requires the manager to balance "tough-love" skills with coaching and leadership. Due to the constant demand for your time and attention, the manager must deal with conflict as soon as it becomes evident, no matter how minor it may seem initially.

The time and effort spent early on will be reflected in staff accountabilities and your having more time to direct your attention to other matters. Conflict will always be in the workplace, people will want to blame someone else, emotions will interfere with judgment, and poor communication skills will interfere with the resolution process. The manager may not be able to change the fact that these challenges exist for them, but the manager can set basic ground rules that clarify for staff the expectations related to their involvement in resolving conflict.

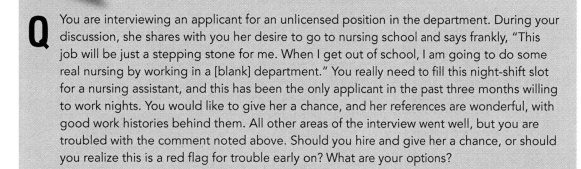

Case Study: An applicant who's ready to move on

Q You are interviewing an applicant for an unlicensed position in the department. During your discussion, she shares with you her desire to go to nursing school and says frankly, "This job will be just a stepping stone for me. When I get out of school, I am going to do some real nursing by working in a [blank] department." You really need to fill this night-shift slot for a nursing assistant, and this has been the only applicant in the past three months willing to work nights. You would like to give her a chance, and her references are wonderful, with good work histories behind them. All other areas of the interview went well, but you are troubled with the comment noted above. Should you hire and give her a chance, or should you realize this is a red flag for trouble early on? What are your options?

A *Discuss this situation with staff and seek their input, especially if you do not have a peer-interview process in place. Share the following with this perspective hire: "I am concerned to hear you say that our department does not have 'real nurses.' Can you explain in more detail what you mean by that? Going to nursing school is an excellent goal, and our facility even has some scholarship programs available that may interest you.*

Should you be selected for this position, my expectation would be that you would be a committed and respectful team member. How do you see yourself doing that if you do not feel this department does 'real nursing?'" Remember, you always have the option to not hire this applicant. Staff may have trouble being short on nights, but that is worth handling instead of having this new hire get on their every last nerve with her attitude toward general nursing.

Recommended reading

1. Buckingham, Marcus and Donald Clifton. Now Discover Your Strengths. New York: Free Press, 2001.

2. Buckingham, Marcus and Kurt Coffman. First Break all the Rules. New York: Simon and Schuster, 1999.

3. Kaye, Beverly, et al. Love 'Em or Lose 'Em. San Francisco: Berrett-Koehler, 1999.

New employee orientation and training

The most important factor in the future success of the new employee is an effective orientation process. Because first impressions are the longest lasting, the manager must plan an orientation program that meets not only the individual needs of the new hire but also the needs of the department or unit. Your goal is to provide all new employees with the tools and resources they need to be successful. Doing so can reduce turnover and prevent staff absenteeism.

Purposes of an orientation program

Before outlining an orientation plan, let's examine the purposes of such a program. A well-developed orientation program ensures that new employees:

- Have the skills and knowledge to perform the requirements of their job descriptions

- Understand how their roles help the organization and the department meet their stated objectives

- Can identify the opportunities for self-improvement available to them

- Feel a sense of pride in their roles and in the organization

- Have all the necessary tools and resources for success

- Experience a transition period to the new work environment

- Understand and have documentation of the manager's expectations of them

Organization-wide orientation

Ensure that the new hire is scheduled for the facility's orientation process, which should include general facility-specific orientation information and an introduction to the nursing department. As a manager, it is your responsibility to ensure that the employee's schedule is arranged so he or she can attend these programs and understands the rationale for them. The orientation plan for acquainting the new employee with the organization should include the following:

1. An explanation of the organizational structure. This should include a session with the chief executive officer (CEO), if possible.

2. A tour of the facility.

3. A review and discussion of its mission/vision statement.

4. The history and background of the organization and its services, plus its plans for the future.

5. An explanation of policies that will affect the employee.

6. An explanation of working conditions, privileges, and duties.

7. Presentation of the employee handbook (if not given at the time of employment).

8. An explanation of rules, regulations, benefits, etc.

9. An explanation of the facility's disaster plan and other required safety training.

10. Introduction to nursing standards related to policy and procedure.

Some elements of orientation will vary by facility practice. Items such as safety issues may be required as part of the departmental orientation. Become familiar with the elements of the facility's orientation process so you can include those elements not covered and avoid duplication of elements already discussed in the departmental orientation.

Departmental orientation

Orientation programs may vary in length and content as well as in how they are delivered. Regardless of their formats, it is imperative that, with any departmental orientation program, the manager institute a method of documenting the new employee's ability to meet all of the requirements of the process. Four months after hire is not the time for you to realize that a basic element of orientation, such as the location of a panic button, was not covered with the employee.

Orientation to the facility or department is not just the responsibility of the manager. In order for the new hire to be successful, staff must be included in this process as well. Just as it takes a village to raise a child, it takes the whole team to embrace and nurture the new hire.

Orientation and regular inservice education

Orientation of your employees may be your most important risk-management tool. When employees are hired, the natural tendency is to try to get them on the schedule as soon as possible, theoretically to save money and ensure that staffing is sufficient. Invest in a solid, thorough orientation program.

This protects the facility legally and ensures the residents receive optimum care. In fact, having a commitment to solid orientation and meaningful, ongoing staff development is an excellent way of reducing the risk of legal exposure. Getting a new job is stressful for everyone, and the stress increases tenfold if the employee is ill-prepared for the position. Explain facility policies during orientation.

Avoid the trap of showing a video or handing the employee a stack of papers to read. Tell them and show them. Augment and reinforce the verbal lessons with audiovisuals. Make sure to provide reference information, such as where additional information and policies and procedures can be located. Upon completion of the orientation, give a written quiz to verify that employees have retained the information. Keep good records of the content presented and employee attendance. Make sure to tell employees how much you value the facility residents and staff. Be sincere! They are your most important assets!

Depending on the position, on-the-job orientation is essential after classroom information is covered. This is a strength in facilities with staff-mentoring programs. Carefully pair the new employee with a staff member who will teach him or her well and set a good example. Ideally, the length of orientation will be based on employee need. We all learn at different rates. Evaluate the new employee's competency and ability to function independently before turning him or her loose. Even highly competent employees will have questions when they begin to work independently. Make sure they have a resource person to turn to. Having a resource person debrief them at the end of each shift for several weeks may also be helpful.

Learning

Action learning occurs when students immediately read, view, and do activities learned in the lesson. This list of teaching methods is not all-inclusive. Your objective should be to recognize that everyone is different, and vary your teaching methods, stimulating as many senses as possible. Remember to apply the old Chinese proverb, "Tell me, I forget. Show me, I remember. Involve me, I understand."

People learn in many different ways. Some use primarily one learning style, and others use a combination of styles. When teaching, try to satisfy as many styles as possible through a variety of creative teaching methods. The visual learner learns by seeing and watching. The auditory learner learns by hearing an explanation of the subject. The cognitive learner learns by reading, studying, then working with the material until he or she figures it out. The kinesthetic learner learns by trial and error.

Importance of follow-up inservice monitoring

Managers are legally responsible for ensuring staff are competent in their responsibilities. Facilities and states interpret the method for verifying staff competence in many different ways. Most facilities complete a written evaluation tool on each staff member annually. These tools evaluate issues such as appearance, attendance, and dependability. Most do not evaluate technical performance or skills used in resident care. Because of this, some facilities verify nursing assistant competency by checking each assistant off on the skills required by the state nursing assistant program.

Some facilities also validate competence and learning after each inservice. They prepare a list of skills or theory information presented, then observe staff performance as unobtrusively as possible to ensure that learning took place. If not, remedial individual or group education is done. These are both excellent methods of verifying staff competence and learning. Whatever method is selected, the facility is responsible for the outcome of the learning and for ensuring the residents receive proper care.

The preceptor

The preceptor is the primary staff member who will assist the new hire through the orientation process. When you match the right preceptor with the new employee, you have the beginnings of a wonderful peer-to-peer working relationship that will set the tone for the rest of the peer group.

If the organization has not already done so, the manager should institute a preceptor program. As you become acquainted with the skill levels and personalities of staff members, it becomes easier to identify those with a potential for precepting new hires. The preceptor should have a job description that defines key characteristics such as the following:

- Enjoys teaching adult learners

- Is enthusiastic about the department and the organization

- Wants to be a part of ensuring that new hires are successful in their jobs

- Displays an eagerness to learn new things and a caring for other team members

- Is capable of effectively communicating constructive criticism

- Is perceived by his or her peer group to be a role model

- Demonstrates the ability to solve problems and handle conflict appropriately

In addition to possessing certain personal characteristics, preceptor candidates must also meet specific skill and performance criteria. A staff member that constantly chooses not to follow policy and procedure, for example, should not be a candidate for the additional role of preceptor. Consider the following when selecting preceptors:

- Do they have a set amount of clinical time/experience in the specialty for which the employee was hired? Staff can decide as a group what this time period should be.

- Is their licensure level appropriate? An RN should oversee orientation of another RN, not of an LPN. However it may be appropriate for a LPN to be used as an assistant preceptor in some areas of the orientation.

- Do they meet the annual requirements for competency renewals?

- Do they display excellent organizational skills during their shift duties?

- Do they participate in educational offerings that are beyond their annual requirements?

- Do they exhibit the ability to apply critical thinking skills to patient care processes?

Once you have identified potential preceptors, meet with them on a regular basis to ensure that:

- They understand the expectations you have of them

- They have all the supplies, resources, and tools they need

- They recognize the importance of their role to the department and the organization

- Their ideas and suggestions for improvement are incorporated into the orientation process

The manager will need to maintain momentum and enthusiasm in the preceptors by demonstrating appreciation and offering them rewards. Consider the following possible rewards:

- Vouchers for food in the cafeteria

- Applying the preceptor role to clinical ladders

- Annual breakfast with the CEO to recognize their efforts

- Additional logo/insignia on name badge that identifies them as a mentor

- Salary adjustment

- Tickets to the local movie theater

- Registration fees for an annual nursing conference

Establishing an environment for transition

Orientation for a new hire is a time of uncertainty—even the most learned adults fear failure in new settings. These fears can interfere with their ability to learn at a pace that is acceptable to the manager or their peer group. With unfamiliar equipment, new policies and procedures, and new telephone extensions to memorize, what may be perceived to be the simplest of tasks can be the most frustrating for the new hire.

This leads to increased stress for the new employee as well as to situations where the new hire pretends to know or understand a task or procedure. To prevent this scenario from occurring and to minimize the stress for the employee, the manager should ensure that the orientation process begins with certain basic elements to make the new hire feels at home while transitioning into this new environment. The manager should ensure that the new employee:

- Meets fellow employees

- Knows where and to whom he or she is to report

- Knows the location of the cafeteria, locker rooms, time clocks, restrooms, etc.

- Knows the exact hours of work and time for rest and meal periods

- Knows the rules and regulations governing the department and its employees

- Understands the dress code and knows where to purchase the required uniforms

- Is shown any and all security devices, such as panic buttons or alarms

- Is given a list of the most common items staff need to access

Consider using a scavenger hunt to teach some of the above items. Having new hires participate in such an activity will prevent a scenario in which they are aimlessly wandering through the department, trying to remember where supplies and equipment are located. With the scavenger hunt, the new hire has a purpose, and this activity also encourages conversation with peer group members as they seek help in finding rooms, supplies, time sheets, etc.

Setting goals and timelines

Orientation should include a session in which the manager, new employee, and his or her preceptor identify short- and long-term goals for the orientation. Adults vary in their ability to learn and retain information, and this element must be taken into consideration when establishing these timelines.

The experience and maturity of the new hire will have a direct effect on the length of time designated for the orientation process. Some organizations define this time for overall orientation and then leave it to the manager to determine a timeline for department-specific orientation. If you decide to predetermine a timeline for your orientation process, be sure to clarify what the process will be for those who cannot meet the timeline. For example, an employee may have an outdated basic life support (BLS) card and may not have access to another course until three weeks after the date by which they are due to complete orientation.

In cases like this one, you can have a general statement that gives the new hire, the preceptor, and the manager flexibility with the timeline. Consider including the following language in your orientation policy:

> The orientation process will be designed to meet the individual learning needs of the new employee. Those who cannot complete the required outcomes during a period of _____ will be considered for an extension if the manager and preceptor feel that the employee can meet the requirements of the job description. Those new employees who meet the required outcomes ahead of schedule may be taken off orientation earlier if the preceptor, manager, and employee agree that they can safely meet and demonstrate the requirements of the job description.

Verifying accountabilities and competencies

To ensure that it is clear what is expected of the new hire and that the orientation process has been successfully completed, the manager needs a process to document not only learning activities but also accountabilities. The employee should be required to sign a form confirming that they have received, and agreed to follow:

- The employee handbook

- The organization's mission statement

- His or her job description

- The orientation requirements

To some managers, this may seem to be overkill or too formal, but when you look at the amount of time and money invested in orientating one staff person, the effort is well worth it.

When dealing with licensed professionals, it is important to realize that it is quite acceptable to hold them accountable to their job requirements, and doing so from day one sets the standard. Some organizations actually use a contract for orientation, which the employee, preceptor, and manager all sign. The contract clarifies each person's roles and responsibilities and may put the new hire more at ease when they see in writing that the preceptor is there to help them, not to test them.

In order to hold new hires accountable to the job requirements, you must have a process for validating their performance on the job skills and tasks (i.e., competencies) expected of them. Validation of these competencies should be recorded on a flow chart that includes the following:

- The skill

- Date it was introduced

- Method used to introduce it (e.g., demonstration, video, discussion, etc.)

- Date new employee demonstrated ability to perform it independently

- Dates of expiration of any required certification (e.g., BLS or advanced cardiac life support (ACLS)), if applicable

- Area to note comments

Make no assumptions during the orientation process, especially during skills assessments. Just because the new hire has been performing a particular task for 12 years does not mean that he or she has been performing it correctly or according to your standards. Everything must be demonstrated, from giving an IM injection to placing a patient on a monitor. Explain to the new hire the rationale for this requirement so they do not become defensive

Defining completion of orientation

Predetermine what your standard is going to be to indicate that the employee has successfully completed the orientation process. Institute with the preceptors a checklist on which they can track these items as they are completed. Items to consider for this checklist include the following:

- Completion of facility and safety orientation

- Completion of nursing orientation

- Verification of status of licensure and certifications required

- New hire accountabilities signed (job description, handbook, etc.)

- Completion of scavenger hunt

- Completion of skills/tasks checklist with preceptor

- Completion of feedback form related to the orientation process

Follow-ups

The orientation program incorporates new employee indoctrination, job training, performance, and follow-up. For the purposes of retention and continued acceptable performance after the formal orientation program, individual periodic follow-up interviews should be conducted for new employees by the manager/preceptor.

The new hire will need redirection and support for a period of time that extends beyond the formal orientation process. You may elect to provide it after the probationary period of hire and then again in three months and six months. Do not wait for a scheduled review process to address concerns.

With the essential elements for success, an attitude that embraces the preceptor process, and the right preceptor, your department will benefit greatly from their presence, as will the new employee. Who knows—maybe the new employee will become your next preceptor. That is how the manager truly can define success for his or her orientation program.

Case Study: **The over-ambitious nursing assistant**

Thomas has recently been hired as a nursing assistant. He is also enrolled as a student at a local nursing school. Three weeks into his orientation program, his preceptor approaches you with some concerns. She has noticed that Thomas is spending more time on observing skills and tasks that align with a nurse's role than those required by his job description. His orientation competency check-off sheets are not being kept up to date, and staff have been grumbling about Thomas' reluctance to perform the duties of a nursing assistant. The preceptor is looking for some guidance from you on how to best handle this situation with Thomas. What should you do?

Remember that your role as manager is to clarify the expectations for Thomas and to ensure that he meets the requirements of the job description for which he was hired. The role of the preceptor is to act as an educator, resource person, and evaluator of a new hire's performance, based on the specific duties outlined in the job description. Schedule a meeting with Thomas and his preceptor. When you all gather, make sure to have a copy of his job description, as well as the orientation contract he signed (if applicable). Explain to Thomas that you find it a valuable asset to have a nursing assistant that is enrolled in nursing school. However, it is a priority that he understand the responsibilities outlined in the job description.

Inquire if he has any questions about the specifics of the job description. If he doesn't, indicate that your expectations are that he will complete his competency sheets in a timely manner and make his preceptor aware of any concerns he has related to his job responsibilities. Encourage him to take advantage of all learning opportunities in the department after he has fulfilled the responsibilities of his job and inquired of the charge nurse whether there are other tasks with which he needs to assist. Specify dates by which you expect his forms to be completed and schedule a follow-up meeting for two weeks from the day of your initial meeting. Conclude the meeting with what your expectations are of his preceptor as well, which will help take the load off of the preceptor for having brought the concern to your attention.

Recommended reading

1. Kaye, Beverly, et al. Love 'Em or Lose 'Em. San Francisco: Berrett-Koehler, 1999.

Time management and delegation

You won't find it in your wallet or your bank account. You can't borrow it. You can't work harder and earn more of it. In fact, all you can do with it is spend it. It's time, of course, the one thing of which every manager wishes they had more.

"Time crooks"

In order for a time management process to work, it is important to know what aspects of our personal time management need to be improved. Below you will find some of the most frequent behaviors that reduce effectiveness in the workplace. Check those that you feel are the major obstacles to your own time management and refer to these as your time crooks.

- ❑ Interruptions from telephone calls
- ❑ Interruptions from personal visitors
- ❑ Meetings
- ❑ Tasks you should have delegated
- ❑ Procrastination and indecision
- ❑ Acting with incomplete information
- ❑ Dealing with employees that display unacceptable behaviors
- ❑ Crisis management
- ❑ Unclear communication
- ❑ Inadequate technical knowledge
- ❑ Unclear objectives and priorities
- ❑ Lack of planning
- ❑ Stress and fatigue
- ❑ Inability to say no
- ❑ Mismanagement of paper flow and personal disorganization

Fortunately, there are strategies you can use to manage your time, feel more in control, and reduce stress. If you stop to analyze how you spend your time, you will identify that you are both the cause of and the solution to your time challenges.

Time management systems

Call it a day timer, a personal data assistant (PDA), a pocket calendar, or anything you want. Bind it, sync it, clip it, staple it, or hook it together—the bottom line is that you need to find a system that works for you and allows you to:

- Maintain a calendar of commitments

- Make notes

- Carry it with you at all times

- Include your business cards

- Access commonly used telephone numbers

But as helpful as these organizers are, if the manager is not skilled in other areas of time management, the tool will not be of any benefit at all. It won't work for a manager who lacks the necessary skills for setting priorities, delegating responsibilities, and confronting procrastination.

When you address and improve these three skills, you find yourself with more time. What other reason do you need to improve your time management behaviors?

Priority setting

You think you've successfully outlined your priorities for the day. But just when you thought it was safe to show up for work, you get to the building, and your staff are lined up at the door waiting for you, your pager is going off, the message light on your voice mail is flashing endlessly, and your inbox is full of e-mails. All of a sudden, your priority list is a vague memory.

This is the point in the day that separates the good managers from the effective managers. Effective management requires you to know when and when not to reshuffle your priorities after you walk into a situation that may take precedence. If there is something that absolutely must be attended to immediately—something that was not on the list you showed up with—someone is going to make you aware of that fact.

Consider asking those waiting in the line if any of them has an emergency that requires your immediate attention. If not, explain that you would be happy to make time for them later in the day, if needed. You should explain that there is already an urgent matter that requires your attention first thing this morning.

"The key is not to prioritize what's on your schedule but to schedule your priorities."

These words by Stephen R. Covey remind us that managers needs to maintain control of determining where to focus their attention next. Don't let the behaviors of others decide this for you. There are a lot of great actors out there who will dramatize scenarios in hopes of getting you to focus your attention on what they believe to be your most important priority. Remember that you are the manager, and the organization expects your priority setting to be done with the best interests of the patient in mind. A helpful priority-setting tool for managers will prompt them to put pen to paper and write out the:

- Function or task

- Deadline date(s)

- Whom it affects

As you schedule your priorities, these types of tools help you focus on where your time is best spent today or right now.

When you feel overwhelmed with priorities, take your spreadsheet to your manager and ask his or her opinion—what does he or she think are the top three things that deserve your time today?

Case study: Early morning priority issues

Q Last night, you received a call at home regarding a resident complaint related to a bad outcome of an error that occurred. Driving in today, you realize that this is a priority for you to address. When you arrive at work, you are faced with a voice mail message from a night shift nurse who is crying on the phone about another incident that occurred last night. He strongly expresses the need to talk with you "first thing this morning." Where is your attention going first?

A *Return the call to the night shift nurse confirming that you did receive his message. Let him know that his issue is important to you and that you plan to give him uninterrupted time to discuss it. Tell him you will call him back today at _____ (time). Ask him if this is a good time for him. Then deal with your original patient-care issue involving the bad outcome. When that is completed, keep your commitment to the nurse and call him back.*

Delegation

Delegation is a means of transferring the responsibility for a procedure or other task from a licensed nurse who is qualified and authorized to perform the activity to another person who does not possess the authority. After a task is delegated, only the person to whom the authority has been given may perform the procedure. This means that this person cannot delegate or assign someone else to do the task. The nurse is accountable for the task and its outcome. He or she does this by first assessing the resident and believing that the resident is stable and the outcome of the activity is predictable. Second, the nurse must be familiar with the scope of practice, qualifications, and competence of the individual to whom the task is being delegated.

In some situations, such as when the resident is unstable, delegation may be inappropriate, even if the task is a simple one. Some states provide further definitions for the terms "delegation" and "assignment." Assigning means advising, instructing, or informing a subordinate to complete a task. The person making the assignment must possess the authority to do so. Delegation is only made to licensed personnel. In states that make a distinction between assignment and delegation, "delegate" means to authorize or entrust another to do the task. The person doing the delegation entrusts another and authorizes him or her to take the responsibility for seeing it is done.

Delegation is a management principle used to obtain desired results through the work of others, and it is a legal concept used to empower one to act for another. Professional skill and expertise in delegation have a positive impact on resident care. Individuals to whom responsibility is delegated must have the ability to accept and perform delegated activities. The outcomes of effective delegation include:

- Allowing protection of resident safety

- Achieving desirable resident outcomes

- Facilitating access to appropriate levels of healthcare

- Delineating the spectrum of accountability for nursing care

- Decreasing nurse liability

Your state board of nursing and the National Council of State Boards of Nursing have delegation guidelines available. Check both sources for a comprehensive overview of nursing responsibilities. The Director of Nursing is responsible for overseeing activities and ensuring that delegation in the nursing department is safe and appropriate.

Five rights of delegation

The National Council of State Boards of Nursing has developed a guide titled *The Five Rights of Delegation*.1 The nurse must verify the delegation is appropriate. Appropriate delegation assures the following:

- The nurse is certain that delegating the activity is not against the law.

- The person to whom the task is delegated has been taught to perform the procedure. He or she can demonstrate the procedure correctly, if necessary.

- The resident is stable, and frequent, repeated assessments are not necessary.

- The resident's response to the activity is reasonably predictable.

- In the nurse's opinion, the person to whom the task is delegated will obtain the same or similar results as the nurse in performing the procedure.

In some situations, delegation is inappropriate. For example, an unstable resident needs the assessment skills of a licensed nurse during a procedure. In this case, the procedure cannot be delegated. Inappropriate delegation of activities that are routinely done by unlicensed personnel provides potential legal problems. Assessment is an activity that cannot be delegated to an LPN or nursing assistant. Part of the assessment consists of organizing, analyzing, prioritizing, evaluating, and synthesizing data. This must be done by an RN. However, other caregivers can assist with the collection of assessment data by obtaining vital signs, height, weight, and other information. The RN will use this information to develop an overall plan. Other caregivers may contribute to the plan, but the responsibility for its development cannot be delegated.

The inability to effectively delegate can be one of the greatest obstacles to time management for any manager. Delegating is the act of empowering and making others accountable. Many managers feel they do a good job of delegating when actually there may be plenty of room for improvement.

Sometimes your attempts to delegate will fail. In these instances, it is important to review the events to identify the obstacle(s) to successful delegating. Common reasons that delegation fails for managers include:

- Not investing enough time up front with the person you are delegating to

- Not giving staff permission to make mistakes when you delegate functions to them

- Having an I'd-rather-do-it-myself attitude

- Control and power issues

- The perception that staff is not qualified to handle the task

Every time the manager decides not to delegate something to staff, that decision sends an unspoken message to employees. Staff are left feeling that you:

- Don't trust them

- Do not recognize their skills and capabilities

- Do not believe they have the capability to learn new things and grow in their roles and are a control freak

When you are in a position to delegate functions or tasks to staff, give them all the important details and encouragement—set up the situation for success. Doing so will make them feel good about participating, and you will feel pride in what they have accomplished.

Tips for delegation success:

- Describe in detail the specifics of what you are delegating

- Be selective about to whom you delegate what

- Delegate small tasks at first

- Be a resource for them without taking over the project

- Give realistic timelines for completion

- Provide them with the tools and resources necessary to complete the task

- Grant the authority and permission for staff to make pertinent decisions

- Reward and recognize their successes in a timely manner

- Clarify your expectations over and over again

Keep in mind, every time you make a decision to delegate and involve staff you are:

- Freeing up time for you to focus on other job duties

- Building staff self-esteem and growing new leaders

- Sending a clear message to staff that teamwork is valued

- Displaying to the organization the level of trust the department has built with you in the lead

However, be careful that you never dump a problem on staff because you are tired of dealing with it—that is inappropriate behavior for a manager. Also avoid letting delegated tasks fall by the wayside. Schedule time with the staff members you've entrusted with a responsibility to review their progress and be a resource for them.

Case Study: A resistant delegate

Q You have delegated specific tasks to staff members based on their individual interests and skills as a way to improve staff involvement and accountabilities. One clerk approaches you, saying that she feels she does her job well and shouldn't have to be doing any of this "extra stuff." "After all," she says, "you're the manager and get paid the big bucks. Why aren't you doing it?" What is the appropriate response?

A *Get copies of your job description and the clerk's job description and call her into a meeting. Highlight the part of her job description that notes "actively participates in_____" and point out to her on your job description the requirement to "oversee staff involvement in_____." Ask whether she has any questions related to those responsibilities and, if not, clarify your expectations of her related to her job description. Keep the conversation short and to the point.*

Confronting procrastination

Procrastination is the art of keeping up with yesterday. It may signal poor delegating skills, lack of a structure for accountability, or fear of facing the consequences of confronting someone or something.

Tasks that managers often procrastinate over include:

- Budget reviews or preparations

- Confrontations with staff regarding unacceptable behaviors

- Annual evaluation reviews of staff

- Administrative reports

- Completion of forms, forms, and more forms

A variety of approaches can help managers with procrastination. The challenge is to find the one that meets your needs and your management style. For some managers, first tackling the items they most commonly procrastinate over works well. For others, scheduling specific times to perform the tasks can be helpful, as long as you agree with yourself not to reschedule it—otherwise, you're procrastinating again.

Before you feel the urge to procrastinate, you need to ask yourself these important questions:

- What will happen if I don't deal with this now/today?

- Will not dealing with this affect others?

- Will not dealing with this affect how my performance is perceived?

Once you recognize that not dealing with an employee's evaluation will affect how quickly he or she gets a raise, you may designate a different level of urgency to this item. Not attending to a budget report may leave the chief financial officer (CFO) with the impression that you feel finances are not important. This could affect communications when you make a case for more departmental full-time employees.

Self-discipline and self-direction are characteristics of effective leaders, and they come in handy when dealing with procrastination. To minimize procrastination:

- Reward yourself when you attend to matters over which you typically procrastinate

- Give yourself a pat on the back and say "good job" to yourself

- When completing these tasks, attend to something you absolutely love about your job, such as spending some time with patients and their families

Are you time-conscious?

The people who get the most done are almost always "time-haunted." Unless you cultivate respect for time and are continually conscious of its passage, you are apt to waste it. The following quiz will give you an idea of how much "time sensitivity" you have.

1. Do you know how much one hour of your time is worth?

2. Is your day's schedule of activities firmly in your mind when you arrive at work?

3. Do you have a fairly accurate idea of what you ought to get done this week? This month? This quarter?

4. Have you delegated as much work as possible?

5. Do you weigh the time requirements of various tasks before assigning them to others or undertaking them yourself?

6. Do you wade right into the high-priority, tough, and unpleasant jobs rather than devoting too much time to the things you like to do?

7. Do you carry a notebook with you for jotting down ideas, important information, sudden insights, etc., rather than relying on your memory?

8. Do you use modern technology to save time (e.g., conference phone calls, computers, etc.)?

9. Is there a steady flow of communications between you and your staff, with a minimum of backtracking, questions, and requests for clarification?

10. Do you consciously appraise—and police—your use of leisure time?

11. Have you developed routine ways of handling routine matters, like correspondence, requests for information, and so on, or does every little thing throw you off base?

12. When things are going exceptionally well, do you take advantage of the psychological momentum by tackling other tough chores, or do you bask in your accomplishment and ease off for the rest of the day or week?

13. Do you ever challenge the way things are done—not because you necessarily have a better idea but simply because you think there is always a more efficient way to get things done?

14. Do you make it a habit to have some fill-in jobs waiting for your attention, just in case you suddenly find yourself with some spare time (e.g., an expected visitor breaks an appointment)?

Scoring: Three or more "no's" suggest that it's time to change your ways.

Managing your time more efficiently

Sometimes the most difficult thing to accomplish at work is work. With telephone calls, meetings, visitors, and faxes, not to mention the deluge of mail, e-mail, and internal memos, it can be almost impossible to get anything done. Here are some tips to help you stay on track:

- Keep a log for a week. As you evaluate the tasks that consume your time, ask yourself: Do I really need to do this? Could I have delayed this task in order to work on a task of higher priority? Could someone else have done this?

- Determine which times of day are your most productive and schedule your most challenging jobs for those times. If you're a morning person, set aside time in the morning; if you come alive after lunch, block out time then.

- Make appointments with yourself. If you have a big project that you need to start, set aside time for it and write it on your calendar.

- Build flexibility into your schedule so you can adapt when things don't go according to schedule or when new opportunities arise.

- Estimate how long you need to finish a certain project; it will help you manage your time. (Always anticipate that projects will take longer than expected.)

- When you return a phone call, minimize phone tag by including a time you can be reached when you leave a message.

- Review tasks to determine whether any of them can be delegated.

- Limit how many times per day you check your e-mail. (Remember, if there is something really pressing, people will find you.)

- Vary your pace. No one can function at top speed all day. After a mentally taxing project, turn to something less demanding. Put small, enjoyable jobs in between tough ones. Also, take breaks to refresh yourself; you'll be more productive.

- Split long tasks into smaller increments to allow you to fit them into available time.

- Divide a difficult job into several parts so you don't burn out before it's done.

- Be decisive, and then implement the decisions you make.

- Expect interruptions. We can learn how to minimize them, but they may be inevitable.

- Assign yourself one task/process to look forward to each day. For example:

  - Spend lunch time with your most motivated employee

  - Cover a patient assignment for 30 minutes while a staff member takes his or her meal break

  - Schedule time with your mentor for some personal coaching opportunities

- Value your time, and ask others to value it, too

- Consider asking your boss to allow you to trial one work day per month at h
  allows you to catch up with paperwork in an environment of fewer interruptic

Recommended reading

1. Blanchard, Ken, et al. Everyone's a Coach. Grand Rapids, MI: Zondervan, 1995.

2. Cannon, Jeff, et al. Leadership Lessons of the Navy Seals. New York: McGraw-Hill, 2003.

3. Glen, Peter. It's Not My Department. New York: Berkley Books, 1990.

4. Rees, Fran. Teamwork from Start to Finish. San Francisco: Pfeiffer, 1997.

5. Robbins, Anthony. Unlimited Power. New York: Fawcett Columbine, 1986.

References

1. National Council of State Boards of Nursing. (1995). Delegation concepts and decision-making process. Online. http://www.ncsbn.org/regulation/uap_delegation_documents_delegation.asp. Accessed 11/04/05.

CHAPTER 8

Conflict resolution/ managing complaints

Working in long-term care

Conflict is an inevitable part of working in long-term care. Staffing, stress, close environments, and rapid decision-making all set the stage for conflict on the nursing units. Since each unit is part of a larger whole and does not operate in a vacuum, conflict may occur between units, and with other departments. Conflicts may also occur with residents and family members. Instead of becoming overwhelmed by complaints and conflicts, view them as wonderful opportunities for making improvements. Doing this takes only a minor attitude adjustment and a slight change in perspective.

One study revealed that nurse managers spent 20% of their time on conflict management tasks. These managers rated conflict resolution skills as being more important than planning, motivation, communication, and decision-making.[1] Interpersonal conflict was a strong predictor of job satisfaction in several studies. Nurses who experienced more interpersonal conflict were often dissatisfied with their jobs.[2,3] Yet another study showed an inverse association between stress and job satisfaction. In this study, job satisfaction was low when stress was high.

Unresolved conflict creates a stressful work environment. Stress also occurs when the workers perceive unreasonable or inappropriate demands on their time, unfair or improper assignments, or conflicting goals and values.[4] One study seemed to suggest that there was a significant difference in the predicted and observed death rate in a facility experiencing intergroup conflict between physicians and nurses. When physicians and nurses disagree, collaboration and creativity are stifled, with an increased risk for poor patient outcomes.[5] Resolving conflict entirely is an admirable goal. If this cannot be achieved, strive for a compromise that everyone can live with, and continue to keep communication open. Properly managed conflict is helpful in improving or changing a facility, making it more efficient and competitive. Although conflict resolution does not always lead to a complete resolution of the problem, the underlying issues must be settled, or the potential for escalating future problems will always exist.

Conflict

Conflict is a normal part of working in long-term care. When issues and priorities collide, conflict usually follows. Differences of opinion are part of life, and are not necessarily bad. In fact, conflict can be healthy, such as when it exposes differences that need to be discussed and resolved. It may mean employees care deeply about an issue. Unfortunately, conflict has the potential to be very divisive. Providing a forum for open and honest conflict resolution can further employee growth. Whether the net effect of workplace conflict is positive or negative is determined by how we respond to it and how it is handled.

To a degree, identifying differences of opinion helps people develop a sense of self. Differences help people learn good communication skills. They help people take responsibility for their feelings and actions. Occasionally, conflict is a motivator, because it connects people with new ideas and other points of view and ways of thinking. However, conflict cannot be ignored. It must be managed so that workers will continue to cooperate to get things done. Handled correctly, interdepartmental conflict can enhance organizational performance and promote teamwork. It may also enhance individual performance. If unresolved conflict is ignored, it may lead to serious organizational dysfunction.

Communicating with others

Teach employees to use tact and sensitivity when communicating with others. The impression you provide can be unintentionally negative. You can be 100% right in your conclusions, reasons, beliefs, and opinions, but 100% wrong in how you express them. People who know they are right are sometimes blunt, arrogant, and offensive. You can be honest without being offensive or brutal. Always treat others, including subordinates, with dignity and respect. Attack an action, if necessary. Avoid attacking a person. Send "I" messages. Use the golden rule. A newer paradigm, the "platinum rule," implies that you should treat others how they want to be treated. The focus of relationships shifts from "This is what I want, so I'll give everyone the same thing" to "Let me first understand what they want and then I'll give it to them."[6] Be assertive, not aggressive. The difference is that assertive individuals are respectful, whereas aggressive individuals are not. In fact, they are often abrasive.

Resolving conflict

Facility management must support conflict resolution at every level. Some facilities have trained and qualified peer mediators in place in each department. You may consider periodic inservices and role-playing activities on communication, conflict management, and conflict resolution to provide staff with useful skills. These are very basic skills that are essential for all workers in the 21st century. A clear understanding of policies, procedures, and addressing conflict is necessary for all employees. The facility should have a systemic mandate and format for addressing conflict in the workplace. Likewise, assertive communication skills are a valuable, yet basic competency. Workers with good communication skills are often viewed as being very effective, compared with others in their position who are less articulate. These workers facilitate positive, respectful communication. They do not come across as being opinionated, abrasive, or offensive. Teach your staff to use "I" messages. These reflect one own feelings, wants, and needs. On the whole, others react with much less resistance and defensiveness to "I" messages than they do to "You" messages, which are often accusatory in tone, even if that is not the speaker's intent. An "I" message has four parts:

- How I feel about this situation

- Actions of others when you _____

- Results of others' behavior on the speaker because _____

- A request for the change I would like

In addition to using "I" messages, conflict can be avoided by:

- Being tolerant and accepting of others

- Respecting the cultural beliefs of others

- Using active listening so others feel as if you understand their position (understanding does not necessarily mean you agree with it)

- Using anger management techniques and positive self-talk, if necessary

- Being assertive

- Proving psychological support to show you understand another's position (being supportive also does not mean you agree with it)

Classifying conflict

There are various descriptions of conflict in healthcare. Conflict normally falls into these categories:

- **Intrapersonal:** Having conflicting feelings about a personal course of action with a resident, family member, or another worker.

- **Interpersonal:** Having recurring differences of opinion with a peer. Occasional differences are healthy and expected. Recurring conflict between the same workers requires further investigation.

- **Intragroup:** In teams of workers on a unit, there are several parties or subgroups conflicting with each other.

- **Intergroup:** This involves an entire team opposing another, such as first-shift workers opposing second-shift workers.

Reasons for conflict

Conflict may occur between employees, between departments, or between resident family members and staff. In long-term care, it often occurs over difference of opinion. It is also commonly caused by:

- Information overload

- Differences in perception or understanding

- Frequent changes in directions, causing confusion

- Inadequate or incorrect information

- Lack of information, misinformation, disagreement about what information is important or what it means

- Disputes over what is needed to meet one's needs.

- Poor communication, personality and behavior clashes

- Stereotyping, cultural or generational differences

- Differing values and ethics (these are among the most difficult to resolve)

- Power struggles, feeling powerless and out of control

- Unequal decision-making ability, power, and control

Other factors that increase stress and lead to conflict in long-term care workers are:

- **Role conflict**—when workers have conflicting loyalties or guidelines, or are expected to do things that contradict their own ethics, values, beliefs, principles, or expectations.

- **Role ambiguity**—when workers do not clearly understand their job description or responsibilities, including what is expected, and limits on their scope of authority.

- **Work overload**—when workers perceive their workload to be too heavy, or feel they are expected to do too much work in too little time.

- **Time pressures**—when workers believe they cannot complete their assigned work within the designated period of time without cutting corners, taking shortcuts, or compromising safety.

- **Low self-esteem/need for self-protection**—workers are insecure and react to past or present conflict by reduced productivity, reduced risk taking to avoid criticism, and blaming others.

- These workers are those who are present in body, but not in spirit. They often take everything personally, and usually feel very anxious and stressed.

The factors listed above can be particularly unnerving for the workers, because, to resolve them, they probably need to meet with a supervisor, whom the worker perceives as unreceptive to the conversation.

Undoubtedly, the worker feels as if he or she is taking a risk. However, managers must be prepared to discuss and negotiate these problems, which will inevitably occur. If nothing else, the supervisor can clarify worker expectations, investigate workload problems, and make adjustments when necessary. He or she may also be able to help the worker improve his or her organizational skills. Good organization is essential in healthcare, but it must be learned in practice, not the classroom. The most successful workers are often those who are well-organized, with good time management skills.

The initial reaction to conflict is commonly influenced by emotion rather than intellect. Because managing conflict involves managing feelings and opinions, it may be difficult to resolve. Resolving conflict in a mature manner within the confines of the facility is always better than resolving it in the courtroom or through a complaint survey. Teach staff to accept conflict and complaints graciously. Avoid becoming defensive because of the complaining party's tone of voice or body language. Listen carefully and respond sincerely and clearly. Monitor your own facial expression and body language. If a resident or family member complains, thank them for notifying you and assure them their concern will be addressed. (Remember to view it as an opportunity for improvement.) A charge nurse or other administrative person should follow up with them later to be sure they are satisfied with the remedy and the outcome.

Coping with conflict

Many people use a variety of coping styles and skills in conflict resolution. However, some have only one style of coping, and use nothing else. Common ways of managing conflict are:

- **Competition**—Being aggressive and uncooperative. This style may be used when a person cares deeply about the problem.

- **Avoidance**—avoiding and refusing to discuss conflict because of fear of expressing it, difficulty articulating the problem, or not really caring about the person or situation.

- **Accommodation**—giving in to others because doing so is easier. People who use this style may build up anger and resentment over time.

- **Collaboration and compromise**—This is the healthiest method of managing conflict, and people who use this style are often confident in their ability to manage it. They know that neither party will have all his or her needs met, and look for mutually beneficial solutions. This style is the most effective in major and complex conflicts in which both sides are committed to finding solutions.

- **Severe reactions**—Many healthcare workers (including nurses) have difficulty handling conflict. Rather than face conflict, employees may call in sick, withdraw, change shifts or assigned areas, resign, or eventually leave long-term care nursing.

Collaboration

Collaboration is the most effective method of conflict resolution. Working together to solve a problem gives staff ownership, which results in a mutual commitment to working things out. To collaborate effectively, personnel meet together and agree to take an open, insightful look at the issues and available resolutions. Collaboration is a team-building skill that proves that working together helps achieve personal and departmental goals. Collaboration decreases stress and improves interpersonal (and interdepartmental) communications. Staff who participate in conflict resolution often gain a perspective of and appreciation for the big picture of facility operations.

Gathering all conflicting parties together and facilitating open communication is one of the best means of resolving the situation amicably. Ignoring conflict only allows it to fester unabated, creating potentially serious circumstances. Begin by informing all involved parties that these are important problems and that you need help and support in figuring out solutions. Before deciding how to intervene, you must identify and understand the problem as fully as possible.

To identify the problem accurately, you must use good communication skills, including active listening. Active listening shows you value the speaker's opinion. Seek to understand the speaker's message; try to understand what he or she wants you to understand. Observe the speaker's content and feeling. Try to identify the issue and restate it. For example, if someone says, "I don't think I can take any more of this," rephrase it by saying, "So you are feeling stressed and overwhelmed." Initially, your role is to listen to and interpret the data. At this juncture, don't do any problem solving. This may be difficult because it involves temporarily giving up control. Concentrate on what is being said and what is going on with people expressing their concerns.

People are responsible and accountable for their own behavior; no one can force another person to swear, become angry, yell, pout, and so forth. Encourage each party to state their goals, feelings, opinions and beliefs without infringing on the rights of others. Set the communication ground rules:

- Identify priorities of individuals in conflict. What do they want to do? What is most important? What needs to be done to make this happen?

- Develop a plan. Set limits on manipulative behavior. This reduces hostility and stress. Reinforce positive behavior; be consistent in setting limits.

Negotiation and conflict management

Many conflicts can be readily managed when issues are accurately identified and defined, then clearly articulated so everyone is on the same page. Begin by trying to accurately identify the origin and source of the conflict. People will probably not thank you for resolving the problem with tact, skill, and diplomacy, but they will undoubtedly remember it if you ignore the problem or manage the situation badly. To solve a problem, you must understand it. Conflict resolutions can be constructive or destructive, depending on the approach. A team approach is a constructive way of resolving conflict. When the team approach is used, outcomes are often better. Poorly managed conflicts cause hurt feelings and negatively affect quality of care. By learning and using negotiation and dispute resolution techniques, your staff can probably resolve many of the interpersonal conflicts that develop each day.

Negotiation is the attempt to reach an agreement or resolution through discussion. Many people view negotiation as a win/lose situation. In other words, the more you get, the less

I get. Try to find a win/win, or mutually acceptable, solution. To do this, you must continue to use active listening skills. You may also have to use the skills of flexibility and persuasion. Be clear in identifying your own needs, or the speaker's needs, while remaining open to the needs of others.

Try to distinguish between demands and needs. To be successful, you must:

- Recognize that a conflict exists; don't ignore it

- Analyze and identify feelings (hurt, anger, jealousy, etc.)

- Separate substantial concerns from interpersonal conflicts

- Accept responsibility for your own behavior and actions

- Plan your strategy

- Describe how you will identify an ongoing problem, recognize it, and measure improvement

- Determine what action you will take if negotiation is not successful

- Set limits; avoid exceeding the limits without first stopping to think it over

The four-C structure may be useful in guiding negotiations:

1. Communicate

2. Clarify

3. Create options

4. Commit to a mutually beneficial resolution

The objective of this communication is to cultivate a stable foundation for discussing the conflict further. Search for areas of agreement, such as identifying common goals. Begin by setting aside a mutually acceptable time and place to meet with all involved parties. Designate the time frame, such as an hour, from the outset and stay with it. Consider using a group activity:

- Have each person write down his or her description of the problem.

- Go around the room, and have each person read aloud what he or she has written.

- Next, ask each person to write down and read aloud "I" messages regarding his or her feelings about the conflict.

- Have each person write down and read aloud what he or she wants and needs and what his or her goals are in relation to the conflict.

- Now do a role reversal. Give each person a time limit to argue an opposing point of view, based on what someone else has said.

- Facilitate the meeting by writing on a flip chart or chalk board. Go around the room and ask each person to share a goal or solution, then list how various goals can be achieved, using compromise if necessary.

- Try to show participants how this is a positive situation. Show how some of each person's needs are met.

- Remain neutral. Avoid passing judgment. Keep the discussion on track and on time.

- Write down a plan of action, including what each person agrees to do, how, and when. Have participants sign at the bottom, if desired.

- The best solution is one that will satisfy the wants and needs of all involved parties. Brainstorming a list of potential solutions, then narrowing it down to those most likely to work, may help.

- After deciding on a course of action, obtain a commitment to the final solution. Ask workers if anything will keep them from fulfilling the agreement. Agree on how the plan will be implemented and set a time for a follow-up meeting to assess progress.

Managerial conflict resolution

There may be times when conflict must be resolved through managerial decision-making, or changes in policies and procedures. Regardless of whether management administers the program or peer mediators are responsible, the formal resolution process must be kept confidential. Accept that you may lose one or more workers after a serious conflict situation, even after the situation has been resolved. When feelings and emotions are involved, people do not forget, especially if they feel wronged. Anticipate that this may occur, and try to take steps to prevent similar problems in the future. When managing conflict:

- Thoroughly investigate and identify the problem.

- Avoid judging. Remain neutral.

- Identify the source of conflict by interviewing everyone who is involved separately.

- Be decisive; keep others informed of the changes to be made, and how outcomes will be measured.

- Always follow up with workers by observation and interview in a reasonable period of time so you are aware of outcomes.

Facility policies

Facility policies should promote conflict management and resolution at all levels. After policies and procedures are in place, give some thought into educating your personnel. Tim Porter-O'Grady has written some excellent articles on this subject. He suggests the following:[7,8]

- Define conflict and explain how it is a normative part of communication.

- List the elements and dynamics of conflict as part of the way humans manage their differences.

- List the basic steps of the conflict resolution process with stages and steps of conflict identified in a systematic problem-solving format.

- Describe the structure and dynamics of the facility's organized conflict resolution process, including methods of access, use, and application to the individual conflict.

- Clearly explain the systematic approaches to resolving conflict as part of the facility's commitment to doing business and resolving problematic issues.

Porter-O'Grady suggests that these elements be included in the formal conflict resolution process (shown in Figure 8-1):

- Welcome, explanation of mediation, explanation of confidential nature of proceedings, ground rules

- Participants' description of the problem, outlining the issues

- Identifying the main concerns, restating the primary issues, writing down the specific understanding related to the issues, reordering the identified primary concerns

- Seeking solutions through participant cooperation, including presenting ideas, brainstorming, and exploration

- Evaluation and selection of ideas for resolution, including priorities of choice, discussing liability, areas of agreement, areas of emerging confluence of solutions

- Enumeration of solutions and specification of impact, response, role, and individual commitment to actions related to solutions

- Documentation of resolution, including all items, performance expectations, follow-up, and evaluation

- Evaluation of the mediation process by participants and mediator

FIGURE 8.1   **Stages of conflict resolution process**

1. Introduction to conflict process

2. Participants' description of situation

3. Identification of core issues

4. Pursuing solutions

5. Evaluation and selection of solutions

6. Agreeing on solutions and actions

7. Documenting agreement and actions

8. Evaluation of mediators and process

State requirements

In some states, facilities are required to have a formal conflict resolution program for use by residents and responsible parties. Figure 8-2 is an example of the requirements for this program in Michigan facilities.

The Michigan model is an example of an excellent process to use. Regardless of the method your facility uses for managing complaints, you may want to consider keeping a complaint log listing at least the:

- Date of initial complaint

FIGURE 8.2   Nursing home resident complaint resolution

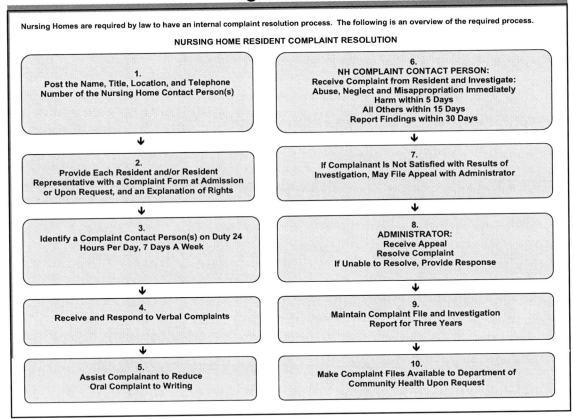

- Summary of complaint

- Name and contact information for individual making the complaint

- Date complaint investigation initiated

- Date and manner of resolution

You may wish to keep a separate file with private details of your investigation, depending on the circumstances of the investigation. When addressing complaints:

- Listen to the complaint

- Repeat or paraphrase to make sure you understand the problem

- Establish the real issue, if possible

- Agree on a resolution

- Agree on a plan of action

- Follow up

References

1. McElhaney, R. (1996). Conflict management in nursing administration. Nursing Management 27. (1996). 49-50.

2. Cox KB. (2003). The effects of intrapersonal, intragroup, and intergroup conflict on team performance effectiveness and work satisfaction. Nurse Admin Q 27; (2); 153-163.

3. Irvine DM, and Evans MG. (1995). Job satisfaction and turnover among nurses: integrating research findings across studies. Nursing Research 44. 1995; 246-253.

4. Blegan MA. (1993). Nurses' job satisfaction: A meta-analysis of related variables. Nursing Research 42. (1993); 36-41.

5. Knaus WA, Wagner DP, Zimmerman JE, Draper EA. (1986). An evaluation of outcome from intensive care in major medical centers. Annals of Internal Medicine, 104, 110-118.

6. Allesandra T. The platinum rule. Online. www.platinumrule.com/aboutpr.asp. Accessed 11/27/05.

7. Porter-O'Grady, T. (2004). Constructing a conflict resolution program for health care. Health Care Manage Rev, 2004, 29 (4), 278-283.

8. Porter-O'Grady, T. (2004). Embracing conflict: Building a healthy community. Health Care Manage Rev, 2004, 29 (3), 181-187.

The disciplinary process and terminations

Managers often dread the issue of discipline due, in part, to the mindset that discipline equals punishment. The first step in dealing effectively with disciplinary issues is to reframe that thinking and instead consider discipline to be an opportunity for solving a situation with a staff member. This process can focus on the problem as a gap between observed behaviors and expected behaviors. Closing this gap requires:

- Problem-solving discussions, not punishment or punitive measures

- Adult interactions rather than parent-child language

- Respect for both the employee and the standards for quality care and teamwork

- Action plans and follow-up

- The employee, not the manager, taking ownership of behavior change

- Playing policeman

Role of the manager

As a manager, you set the tone for the work culture of your unit. If you raise or lower the bar, the staff will meet it. Therefore, managers must walk the talk of the standards conveyed to staff, and their actions must be grounded in the responsibility to ensure quality care and professional behavior for residents, coworkers, and the organization as a whole.

Remembering the responsibility you have to residents and staff can often remove any reluctance you have to dealing with a disciplinary issue. Equally important is the need to respect the staff member involved in a disciplinary issue by:

- Focusing the discussion on the behavior, not the person

- Listening to the staff member's perspective

- Abiding by the HR-established guidelines for fair and equitable treatment

- Discussing the issues in a clear, honest, and direct manner

- Being consistent and following through on agreements made

As disciplinary issues arise, make a point of working in close contact with the employee relations manager. Use this colleague as a coach and discuss any past history, related events, and reservations or concerns you might have about how to talk with the staff member involved. Also, familiarize yourself with the policies, guidelines, and forms that the employee relations manager offers. This is important in assuring that your actions are thought out, fair, and legally defensible.

Preparation is paramount

To prepare yourself for dealing with a disciplinary issue, think through your answers to the following questions:

- Can I explain the gap between expected and observed behaviors?

- Do I have examples that allow me to be specific rather than generalize?

- Am I clear about why this behavior is a problem and needs to change?

- What logical consequences will occur if the behaviors are unchanged?

- What action is needed on my part to deal with this issue? (A comment or coaching? A private, face-to-face meeting? A written warning for the employee's file?)

- Do I have with me the written guidelines that reflect the validation for this disciplinary process (e.g., employee handbook, job description, etc.)?

Take time to think about the answers to these questions and to take notes. Your answers will allow you to notice where you may need to collect additional data, review guidelines from HR, or discuss your thoughts with another manager or the person to whom you report so that you feel clear and organized prior to the one-on-one meeting with your staff member. If there is an emotional component that could cloud the issue or deflect the conversation, then you may want to role-play the conversation with another manager to get the emotion out of the issue and clarify your thinking and your presentation of the issue.

Framework for discussion

Consider the questions you asked yourself and use the following as a framework for talking with the employee:

- Describe the gap in performance—offer examples to clarify

- Listen to the employee's point of view

- Gain agreement on what needs to change and why

- Listen to the steps identified by the employee to take ownership of behavioral change and include ways you intend to support and follow up on this plan

- Review logical consequences that will occur if gap is not closed

Additional points to consider:

- If the meeting becomes emotionally charged and unproductive, then postpone the discussion.

- "This meeting is not filling our needs for problem solving the issues, so I would like to postpone this discussion until later this week and give us time to regroup and come back together in a more productive way." Don't assign blame or resort to parent-child punitive language.

- Listen to the employee with an open mind—remember the truism, "People will shift in their behavior if they feel heard. They will not shift if they don't feel heard."

- Don't be reluctant to admit a mistake and apologize, when appropriate.

Employee discipline

Employees are accountable for following facility policies and procedures. Your policies should include a progressive discipline policy for infractions of various rules. A progressive discipline policy usually begins with an oral warning, then progresses to a series of written warnings, suspension, and termination for policy violations. Allegations of abuse and theft often bypass the mechanisms of the progressive discipline policy because of the potential severity of the offense and risks associated with allowing the employee to remain on duty. In this instance, the person in charge has the authority to suspend the employee without pay until the allegations have been thoroughly investigated.

Other violations, such as "no call, no show" behavior may be considered and written up as a voluntary termination instead of a deviation from the attendance policies. (However, employees should be informed of this procedure in advance.) In any event, facility policies should address discipline, and employees must be aware of policies, procedures, and the penalties for violations.

Oral and written warnings

Your human resources department most probably has a tool to use for documenting employee discipline. One of the most effective is a one-page template on two-copy no carbon required paper. This enables the supervisor to retain the original and give the employee a copy for his or her records. This format may also be used to maintain a record of oral warnings, or another format may be used. Employees are usually not receptive to receiving a "write up," and may be so defensive that any opportunities for teaching and performance improvement are lost.

Some facilities use other terminology for the discipline process, such as "employee memorandum" or "teachable moment." Although these are documented in the same manner as any other progressive discipline, the terminology is more aesthetically acceptable and does not conjure up as many negative emotions.

When issuing a written warning, be as specific as possible. Identify the policy infraction. Objectively state how the employee violated this policy. You may also wish to list corrective action to take, or consequences if the employee violates the policy again. Present the warning to the employee in a private area. Always praise in public, and counsel or discipline in private. Remember to criticize the employee's action, not the person.

Tell the employee that you value him or her and will provide an opportunity to correct the behavior. Verbally state the consequences if the problem persists. Sign and date the warning. Ask the employee to sign the warning. If he or she refuses or disagrees with the warning, document the refusal to sign. Invite the employee to state the disagreement at the bottom of the warning. Give him or her a copy.

Discharge

Termination meetings will be stressful and emotional, but there are ways to make the termination less difficult. A private meeting is probably the best way to handle most employee terminations. Here are some suggestions to consider:

- Take as much time to fire as you did to hire.

- Never terminate in a hurry, especially when you are angry. Take your time and plan both the firing decision and the means by which to carry it out.

Employee termination is a sensitive, difficult task for most managers—rightfully, it should be. Use your written warning form as a precursor to termination. Follow your policies for an aggregate of offenses. For example, as a manager you should be aware of how the progressive policy is implemented. Most facilities require several infractions of the same policy before termination occurs.

Thus, the employee could theoretically receive three warnings about tardiness, three about attendance, and three for violating the smoking policy before termination occurs for any of these offenses. One violation for tardiness, one for attendance, and one for improper smoking does not warrant termination in most facilities. However, you must know how your facility policies are interpreted before proceeding. In some facilities, the administrator or human resources director must approve all terminations. Know and follow your facility policies. Remember that your employees are your greatest asset. Salvaging/retraining them is often preferable to termination and the potential backlash that may occur as a result.

Although some view employee termination as the final step in the disciplinary process, it can better be described as the failure of the disciplinary process to get the employee's attention. Whether the system relies on the traditional approach of verbal and written warnings followed by suspension and termination or a more progressive approach of oral and written reminders followed by a decision-making leave, either approach may fail and require termination.

To prepare for the termination process, imagine yourself defending your actions in court, where you need to prove that your actions were fair and consistent. Talk with HR representatives to be sure you are following guidelines and not jeopardizing your case in any way. Below is a sampling of the kinds of questions you should ask to ensure that you are on solid ground with this decision:

1. Does the termination violate discrimination laws or other federal, state, or local statutes?

2. Is the reason for firing in line with the organization's policies and procedures?

3. Have any assurances, written or oral, been given to the employee about length of employment or job security?

4. Has the reason for discharge happened in the past, and have other employees been handled in a similar manner?

5. How long has the employee worked for the company, and how does the reason for termination stack up against the employee's overall performance record?

6. Has the reason for discharge been progressively documented in the employee's performance review?

7. Has the employee been informed of substandard performance, violation of policies, or other conduct that could lead to termination? Have oral and written reminders and disciplinary actions been adequately documented?

8. Has the employee had an opportunity to correct the problem behavior? Has the employee been told that failure to correct the problem behavior could result in termination?

9. Has the employee been given the opportunity to present his or her side of the story? Are there any extenuating circumstances that might explain substandard performance or misconduct and alter the decision to terminate?

10. Is the employee about to receive financial benefits, like a pension, that will be lessened or eliminated if the employee is terminated?

Document performance to support the decision.

Hopefully you have good documentation procedures in place already and have given the employee evaluations and reminders or a decision-making leave regarding his or her subpar performance.

Consider the timing.

Holding the meeting at the end of the day or during the time just prior to lunch allows for a more graceful exit. Avoid terminating employees on Fridays, as doing so limits the opportunity for job searching or unemployment filing—which will only encourage sulking and recriminations during the weekend.

Draft an outline.

Construct a list of topics that must be covered during the meeting, and follow it carefully so that the emotion of the situation does not take you off track.

Treat the employee with dignity.

Keep in mind that termination is an emotional event, and make every effort to respect the employee's feelings and deal with them in a respectful manner.

Arrange for another employer representative to be present.

Follow the guidelines established by your HR policies for this process, and consult the hospital attorney if you have additional questions that are not addressed in the policy. If the termination is later legally challenged, you'll appreciate having verification of the events during the meeting. It is often advisable to have a male-female team to deal with the actual termination proceedings.

Conduct the meeting at a time and in a place that protects the employee's privacy.

It should be held in a neutral setting, if possible; never in front of other employees; and with no interruptions allowed. Keep it brief. Although it is important to take the appropriate time to prepare and deliver this message, this meeting is not a time for apology or lengthy explanations. If the progressive disciplinary process has been adhered to, the employee knows there has been a problem, despite possible denials. Explain the termination decision as briefly as possible without apologizing for it. Be clear that the decision is final and not negotiable.

Also, be aware that post termination defamation or discrimination claims can be very expensive. Keep the circumstances of the termination confidential and instruct all others to do the same.

Exit interviews

Your facility policies should state your expectations for notice of resignation. Most facilities require notice equivalent to the length of one pay period for direct-care staff, and two pay periods for managers and department heads. Make sure employees are familiar with these requirements. Exit interviews are an excellent method of obtaining employee feedback, along with employee satisfaction surveys.

Unfortunately, this valuable tool is often overlooked in long-term care. Besides obtaining information about the reasons for termination, the interview is also a valuable tool that provides insight into what it takes to do the job. When done correctly, an exit interview is mutually beneficial for both the facility and the former employee. The facility retains and uses the employee's knowledge. The employee can articulate his or her unique contributions, and leave his or her mark.

Exit interviews can be conducted over the phone, in person, over the Internet, or by using a written questionnaire. However, the return rate is not usually as good when you depend upon the employee to complete and mail or email a written survey. Make it clear to the employee who will use the exit interview information and how it will be used. Explain that the purpose of the interview is to collect information that the facility will use.

Employees may be more likely to participate and may be more honest when someone who is not connected with the employer asks the questions. Another alternative is to have a department head from another department or a member of the employee attendance committee conduct the interview. Whoever conducts the interview should be taught to do it properly, however. A nursing assistant may say he or she is leaving for higher pay. What the employee really means is, "You can't pay me enough to work for that charge nurse." Employees tend to identify tangibles, such as salary because they are easier to discuss than intangibles, such as feelings and emotions. The interviewer should be skilled in drawing the employee out.

Study the data collected at exit interviews. Look for trends in age, length of employment, position, assignment, and other variables. Use the information to examine hiring patterns and trends, and to benefit existing and future employees of the facility.

Employee dissatisfaction and retaliation

Sadly, current and former employees sometimes retaliate against the facility for real or perceived slights. Their actions vary widely from doing things such as causing all the care plans to disappear to calling the state hotline and making complaints. Disgruntled employees or former employees may speak negatively about the facility in the community, making remarks such as, "I wouldn't admit my dog to that facility."

Poor leadership may exacerbate work-related stress by isolating individuals and denying access to social support. Managers who have a tendency to be abusive, aggressive, or punitive, and those who lack appropriate leadership skills, increase employee stress.[1] The authors of one study describe the lack of leadership skills in this type of manager as "passive leadership." This management style is a combination of the "laissez-faire" and "management-by-exception" styles of transformational leadership. Those applying the management-by-exception (passive) style ignore problems until the problems are either brought to their attention or become serious enough to demand action.

Managers using the laissez-faire style avoid decision making and the responsibilities associated with their position. Control, autonomy, and decision-making latitude have been identified as factors that affect positive (or conversely, negative) job performance. For many years, researchers have identified control as being the most critical element in promoting positive performance and worker mental health.[2]

Karasek and Theorell assert that a healthy workplace is one in which the worker's level of demand on the job is met with appropriate levels of control, promoting growth and development. Conversely, a job in which demands are high and control is low is theorized to cause stress and burnout.[3]

Obviously, the ideal solution is to manage the facility correctly to prevent conditions from deteriorating in the first place. However, you may be a new manager who inherited a mess from someone else. In this situation, the facility probably has a history of one or more managers using aggressive behavior as a means of controlling subordinates. Your only option is to try to identify and correct the problems, and this is seldom easy. Conditions cannot be changed overnight. One thing is certain: disgruntled, dysfunctional employees are your worst enemy. They are sabotaging the facility internally and in the community. The situation cannot be ignored. Use the progressive discipline process to manage individual problems until a more satisfactory, global solution has been implemented.

Safety considerations

Not everyone deals with the confrontation of termination in an appropriate manner. Never assume that an employee is not one to act out. Consider these safety tips:

- During the meeting, position yourself in a chair at an exit point—not behind a desk, where you have no escape.

- If the employee has demonstrated poor control in the past, insist that another person be present, and be very up front with the employee as to why that person is there.

- Although you don't want to rush through a termination, do not allow the employee to make you repeat the same information over and over. Conclude the meeting and always stay in control.

- Have a process organized prior to your meeting that requires the employee to hand over facility property, keys, badges, etc.

- Be sure that your organization's information systems specialists immediately remove the employee from computer entry in the medication, patient record, lab, and any other electronic format of documentation.

- Inform staff of the termination. Do not make them find out from someone else. Although you can't keep that person from coming onto the property to use the services, you can keep them from coming into the department or staff lounge area to talk with staff.

Case Study: Listening in on a disciplinary meeting

Manager: "Kaye, I wanted to talk with you about a concern I have regarding your relationship with our new grads."

Staff: "I am not aware of any problem—what's the issue?"

Manager: "We have stressed the importance of welcoming new grads and supporting them to improve retention, and yet I get feedback about your being disrespectful to orientees and being critical of them in front of their peers. I thought you were on board with our retention efforts, so I just need to understand your thoughts and see how we can get together on this important issue."

Staff: "I can't recall any time when I behaved that way, and I have made every effort to help these new people. They have so many questions, and sometimes when we are in rush to finish a report I may sound blunt to them, but I am just trying to see that the report ends on time. They don't seem to use their preceptors as well as they could and, as a result, the rest of us get behind when we try to deal with their questions. I think you are blowing this out of proportion. It's not that big of a deal."

Manager: "I need you to know that one of the orientees was in tears in my office last week after being in report with you. She asked to move to another shift so that she would not have to work with you. I asked her to talk with you, but she said that you were so intimidating that she would need to work up her courage to talk with you. Sue, our facility educator, shared with me that she had talked with you about the way you were dealing with these new grads in report and told you about three occasions on which she had observed caustic remarks and put-downs. We also got notice from HR this week that one of the new folks on nights has resigned after just four months, and she stated in her exit interview that she was tired of you humiliating her in report. Her resignation is costly to us in many ways, since we have spent a good deal of time and effort to get her oriented—about $45,000 in replacement costs, to be exact. So it is a big deal, and I need for you to work with me on this and take the issue seriously."

Staff: "I am just trying to give these new people some feedback. I don't mean for it to come across as a put-down."

Manager: "You may see it as feedback, but they hear it as a put-down, and you know perceptions are reality, up to a point."

Staff: "Why don't they come talk to me, instead of running to you or just quitting?"

Manager: "I have asked them to talk with you, but right now I am talking with you, and I need your agreement that we have to close this gap and all get behind a strong push for retention of new grads. What would it look like if you really got behind this effort and worked on how you come across to new grads?"

Staff: "I will try to find some time to talk with Sue and see if the preceptors could be more available to these folks. I can make some time to give them feedback on a one-on-one basis after report. They may be a little later getting out of here if we take time to talk, but that's doable. When I talk with Sue, maybe she could give me some coaching on giving feedback. I know she works with the preceptors on how to do that, and I think there is a video she uses that I could review, too."

Manager: "She may have some books that would be helpful to you as well as you work on how you come across to coworkers."

Staff: "I am not sure when we could find the time for that, but I will get back to you on the idea."

Manager: "When can I expect to hear from you on that meeting?"

Staff: "I will leave Sue a note and get back to you by Friday to let you know when we will meet."

Manager: "Assuming that you can meet in the next two weeks, how about giving me an update on the outcome of your meeting two weeks from Monday? I would also like to talk with you and Sue together once a month for the next few months, just to follow up and see how your plan is working."

Staff: "I am fine with that."

Manager: "I appreciate your willingness to take these steps, and I trust that this oral reminder will be all that is needed to get the situation turned around. You need to know that the choices you make in taking ownership for these changes will influence the choices I will then have to make regarding whether or not to move into a formal disciplinary process, which could include a written reminder. I hope that we can avoid that by having you follow through on your plan and stick with it over time. I look forward to some good feedback next time I meet with the orientees."

Staff: "I am not the bear they think I am, and I will prove that to you and to them."

Key themes:
 Get to the point
 Take time to listen
 Be specific about needed changes
 Gain agreement on an action plan
 Review the follow-up steps
 In discussion, indicate "oral reminder" and follow-up memo

Recommended reading

1. Grote, Dick. Discipline Without Punishment. New York: ANACOM, 1995.

2. Miller, John. QBQ—The Question Behind the Question. Denver: Denver Press, 2001.

References

1. Kelloway, E.K., Sivanathan, N., (MSc Graduate) Francis, L., & Barling, J. (2005). Poor leadership. In J. Barling, E.K. Kelloway, & M. Frone (2005) (Eds.) Handbook of work stress (pp. 89-112) CA: Sage Publications.

2. Hackman, J. R., & Oldham, G. R. (1980). Work redesign. Reading, MA: Addison-Wesley.

3. Karasek, R., & Theorell, T. (1990). Healthy work: Stress, productivity and the reconstruction of working life. New York: Basic Books.

Assessing competencies

An effective competency assessment program is not only key to complying with the Joint Commission's competency-related standards but is also necessary for risk management and for validating staff's ability to meet their job descriptions. Your department's program should focus on verifying and validating the skills and abilities of staff to ensure that they meet the organization's standards. Doing so not only fulfills compliance requirements and validates the knowledge and skills of staff but also contributes to the quality of patient/family services. Competencies must be assessed:

- Before the employee is hired (initial competency assessment)

- During orientation (verification and validation)

- Every year after orientation (annual competency assessment)

Other situations may also require a review of competency, such as a change in policy, procedure, or evidence-based practice information. Your challenge is to keep the process manageable while still meeting the needs of staff and the organization.

Types of competencies

Competency is the demonstration of one or more skills based on knowledge derived from educational programs and experience. It is also the demonstration of appropriate behaviors, such as those related to customer service. Competencies may belong to one or more of the following categories:

- **General**—competencies everyone in the organization must have, such as codes for fire or a severe weather threat, appropriate methods for reporting a medication error, or maintaining a current basic life services (BLS) card.

- **Department-specific**—competencies identified to evaluate and measure all department personnel with regard to their performance of important tasks and functions of the department.

- **Job-specific**—competencies that are specific to a particular position. They define tasks and skills designed as responsibilities of only one position or of a group of similar positions within the department (they may or may not be applicable to all positions in that department).

Joint Commission standards

The Joint Commission's HR standards provide a framework for a competency program and guide HR department personnel and department managers in identifying some of the necessary components of a compliant program.

- HR.3 requires leaders to ensure that the organization assesses, maintains, and continuously improves competency for all staff.

- HR.4 requires managers to ensure staff competency through orientation, ongoing education, and staff demonstration of the skills they have learned.

- HR.5 requires evaluation of staff performance through measurements of department-specific, job-specific, and age-specific competencies.

Although it is vital to ensure compliance with the Joint Commission's requirements, the manager should realize that even if this agency did not exist, competency review and assessment would still be necessary in the healthcare setting.

Choosing competencies to be assessed

Selecting the competencies to assess and evaluate requires the manager to consider:

- The requirements of state boards related to licensed staff

- The Joint Commission's requirements

- Changes in practice related to evidence-based data

- Job descriptions

- The department's educational needs

- Employees' needs

- New technology

- Types of high-volume, low-volume/high-risk, or problem-prone activities (see below)

Elements of competency assessment for orientation should vary greatly from those required in an annual review. At the time of hire and orientation, you will need to verify all of the tasks and skills the employee will be required to perform per their job description. The ongoing and the annual reviews of competency should not repeat the orientation process but should encompass elements such as:

- New equipment and technology in the department

- Changes in a policy or procedure

- Areas of concern identified by resident outcomes or quality review

- New practices related to resident care

- Age-specific criteria as they relate to any of the above

The department should proactively identify those areas they feel to be high-volume duties, low-volume/high-risk duties, and problem-prone duties. Problem-prone duties are frequently or infrequently performed tasks that require troubleshooting skills. Examples include responding to IV pump alarms, using IV contrast dye in the radiology department, and responding to adverse reactions.

The definition of these high-risk, low-volume and problem-prone duties will vary by facility. The role of the manager includes helping staff identify what belongs in these categories as well as ensuring that they understand their definitions. The risk manager of the organization plays an important role in identifying both, as do those employees involved in quality review. Work with these individuals to ensure that you address the appropriate areas of actual and potential concern.

Staff accountabilities

The manager needs to create a process that promotes accountability on the part of employees in order to ensure their participation in the competency review process and that they maintain the level of skill demonstrated or observed. To make certain that staff maintain the skills they have learned in training, review material from a training session, such as how to use certain pieces of new equipment, or review an infrequently performed procedure on a monthly basis, such as inserting temporary pacemakers. However, the manager is not responsible for reminding employees that their competency requirement for using a Glucometer is overdue for renewal. Although you may be responsible for communicating the date and time of the education session for them to attend, showing up is their responsibility.

For the manager, the job description plays an important role in helping staff understand the expectations of their competency. A statement in the job description should hold them accountable to the competency measurement process. When dealing with staff who hold individual licenses for their roles, the manager will find it very helpful to have a copy of the state's Nurse Practice Act with the section noting competency requirements highlighted.

As with any other issues related to noncompliance with job descriptions, those staff who elect not to comply with competency requirements should understand the repercussions of their decisions. Staff cannot pick and choose which competencies they are going to participate in and complete that's your job. They need to understand the seriousness of not attending or completing any of these requirements—and, likewise, the manager cannot pick and choose which ones warrant confrontation with the employee. All competency requirements should be viewed as equally important.

Age-specific competencies

Age-specific competencies are those that account for the different physiological and psychological needs appropriate to the age and developmental stage of your patient population. The demonstration and documentation of age-specific competencies are expected by The Joint Commission. When assessing the adequacy of age-specific care, surveyors will look for proof that staff members are competent to care for their patients.

You do not need a special or separate competency process to validate that you determine staff's ability to apply the skill or task based on the age-specific needs of the patient. For each skill or task that is addressed for competency, however, be sure to include information related to how this task would be done differently for each age group represented in your patient population (which also means that if the department does not care for pediatric patients, then it would not be necessary to assess that aspect of the performance).

Three dimensions of competencies

Managers must ensure that the methods they use to validate competencies accounts for the following three dimensions of competency:

Critical thinking dimension: The critical thinking dimension is the ability to use information or knowledge. It involves more than retaining facts: It demonstrates the employee's ability to apply the knowledge to a situation. It includes skills such as:

- Problem solving

- Time management

- Planning

- Fiscal responsibility

- Clinical reasoning

- Change management

Interpersonal dimension: The interpersonal dimension is the ability to work with others. It includes:

- Communication

- Customer service

- Conflict management

- Working on a team

- Understanding diversity

Technical dimension: The technical dimension involves both knowledge about a particular topic and the ability to perform fine and gross motor functions. It includes:

- Cognitive abilities

- Knowledge (i.e., learned facts)

- Psychomotor ability (e.g., the ability to operate equipment)

- Technical understanding (e.g., how to program an infusion pump)

It is important to choose a validation methodology that evaluates all of the appropriate dimensions. For example, a validation process that only assesses staff's possession of a certain knowledge/skill will tell a manager little about the employee's ability to communicate with multigenerational or culturally diverse populations.

Validation methodologies

You can use a variety of validation methodologies to evaluate competencies. There are at least six different methodologies, each of which specializes in verifying certain types of job skills. Validation methodologies include:

1. Posttest

2. Demonstration/observation

3. Case study/discussion

4. Exemplar

5. Peer review

6. Self-assessment

Using a combination of these methods not only generates more interest among staff but also provides the manager with a true sense of the level of competence at which staff are performing. We all know of people who "test well" but who, when it comes time to actually perform what they were tested on, cannot meet the performance requirements. By allowing staff to participate in various methods of validation, the manager creates a process that will better meet the needs of the patients as well as those of staff.

These methodologies are some of the means an organization or department uses to verify that every staff member is competent in performing the skill sets expected of them and stated in their respective job descriptions. Identify the skill set for each job in your facility and incorporate that skill set into the job description. Because staff are more familiar with their jobs than anyone else is, include them in this process as well.

Six methodologies

1. Posttest—A posttest is a tool used after a training session to evaluate how much information an employee has retained. Posttests can take the form of written tests, puzzles, or games (e.g., Bingo). They evaluate the technical dimension of a skill, task, or activity.

2. Return demonstration/observation of work—In return demonstrations, employees are asked to show how they performed a skill or task after learning the correct technique. They can demonstrate their knowledge in the actual work environment or in a simulated environment, such as a skills lab or computer lab. Observation of work is a technique that managers use to review employee work during their shifts. This technique is best used for employees that produce something (e.g., creating a spreadsheet, making a bed, etc.). In both of these methods, the manager can use a checklist or a self-directed test to validate that an employee has performed the required/standard steps involved in the competency.

3. Case study/discussion group—Case studies or discussion groups (case studies discussed in a group setting) are ideal for validating the critical thinking and interpersonal dimensions. The manager presents a case scenario and asks the employees either to respond to questions in writing or to discuss:

- The decisions they would make or the action(s) they would take if faced with the same scenario

- Their rationale(s) for the action(s) they selected

- Why they did not choose other courses of action

Rather than listen for one correct answer, the manager or facilitator evaluates each employee's ability to apply knowledge, think critically, and solve problems.

4. Exemplars—Exemplars are case studies done in reverse. A manager or facilitator identifies the competency being assessed, and staff provide an actual situation in which they demonstrated that competency. The discussion should follow the same format as case studies/discussion groups (see above).

5. Peer review—In peer review, the manager assesses competencies by obtaining input from other employees who perform the same job. The peer review tool typically is a written form containing attributes or behaviors consistent with organizational policy, standards, etc. Reviewers complete the form and, using a Likert scale (a rating scale, ranging from a response of five, indicating strong agreement, to a response of one, indicating strong disagreement), rate the employee on each statement. The success of this method will depend on the staff having had training on how to conduct peer reviews and their experience with this process.

6. Self-assessment—A self-assessment is a means by which employees assess their own abilities to meet the competency requirements of their job. It should not be used to validate psychomotor skills (i.e., tasks associated with a new piece of equipment). In this method, an employee typically completes a written exercise that his or her manager has developed. The exercise might be a series of statements with which the employee must agree or disagree. Such a tool becomes beneficial when setting annual goals with employees.

This validation methodology cannot be used alone. It would be effective, however, if used along with a peer-review session. A manager could use the two techniques to identify incongruities in an individual's beliefs and values and a peer's observation of how the person actually behaves in a situation.

When do you need to assess staff competencies?

1. Initial competency assessment

Initial competency assessment determines whether the applicant has the proper credentials to perform the responsibilities and duties of the position. The manager needs to ensure that the employee meets the competency requirements by validating education, licensure, and any required registration or certification, etc. In some organizations, this task is completed by the HR department, but even in these situations, the manager should still review the information collected by HR.

2. Verification and validation

Verification and validation occur throughout the employee's orientation and help ensure a consistent level of performance in your department. Before assigning new employees to tasks and duties, they must be prepared to perform them in accordance with the policies and procedures of the organization and the department.

3. Annual competency assessment

All staff should be involved in the process of determining appropriate elements for the annual review. The content should vary each year and comprise selected skills, duties, tasks, and behaviors that reflect:

- Results of performance improvement activities

- Infection-control reviews

- Risk-management reviews

- Additions of new technology

- Needs identified by medical staff or other employees

Successful competency programs

The success of your competency process will depend on the following:

- Are the competencies being assessed relevant to job descriptions?

- Is staff accountability clearly defined? In writing?

- Are you displaying overt support for the process as well as participating in it?

- For those who choose not to meet the competency requirements, have the consequences been made clear?

- Is staff actively participating in the process?

- Is the content of validation being used to educate and motivate staff?

Competency assessment is an ongoing, daily process, and the manager is responsible for instituting a procedure that staff can follow when they observe an employee not performing or behaving according to the defined competency. The procedure should ensure that those who do not comply (e.g., not wearing gloves when they draw blood) do not feel like someone is "telling" on them. This requires an educational process and role playing to teach staff options in approaching one another as well as in reporting noncompliance when necessary.

Manager competency

Competency assessment is not just for staff. Managers must own their competencies as well. If the organization does not have a formal competency process for the management team:

- Review your job description annually for requirements related to licensure, certifications, education, etc.

- Determine whether you are providing any direct patient care at all and, if so, identify a process by which to ensure that your competencies are validated in the same manner as staff's are

- Identify any new forms, procedures, and processes for which you are now responsible and document the name of the person who trained you and the date on which you were trained

Performance evaluations

An important aspect of your role as a manager is not only to motivate staff to meet the requirements of their job but to also hold them accountable for those requirements. The performance evaluation allows both the employee and the manager to:

- Identify performance strengths

- Identify areas that need improvement

- Develop a plan to improve those areas that need improvement

- Review previous unacceptable behaviors and clarify employee status related to them

- Identify short- and long-term career goals

- Have an opportunity for discussion regarding how employees and their roles fit into the needs of the organization and the department

- Exchange information on the specifics of improving the general quality of care delivered in the department

- Provide a documented record of these events that clarifies, in writing, the expectations of both parties

Observation notes

The evaluation process is not a once-a-year meeting; it is ongoing and encompasses direct observation by the manager as well as feedback from the peer group and other department employees. To ensure a successful evaluation process, managers need to develop a system that allows them to keep notes throughout the year related to:

- Employee strengths displayed (e.g., committee involvement)

- Specific dates/times of unacceptable behaviors

- Tardiness

- Complaints from peers

- Errors in performance

- Out-of-dress-code instances

- Attendance at staff meetings and educational sessions

These notes could be kept in your day timer, on index cards kept in a box, or even in a computer spreadsheet that includes staff names and the items you are tracking. Most importantly, when you walk by and see a staff member doing something wonderful for a patient, family, or team member, remember to note it on a pad in your pocket or day timer, and then transfer the information to whatever tracking system you decide to use. If you do not get in the habit of doing this, you will wish you had when evaluation time comes. For instance, if on June 3 at 4:45 p.m. you discuss with a staff member his or her unacceptable use of down time and you don't document it, you will have a harder time validating your position when you try to address this issue during the evaluation.

Preparing for the evaluation

Lack of preparation will diminish the effectiveness of the evaluation process and will heighten the stress on the manager and the staff member. The time you spend preparing will offset the time you would spend during and after the evaluation trying to validate the comments and expectations you have shared with the employee.

Although much of the preparation is paper-based, some of it also involves mental preparation on the part of the manager. Keep the following in mind:

- Feel confident knowing that you have the necessary documentation to support the comments you will be sharing with the employee.

- The expectations come from the organization, and you are delivering the message on its behalf.

- It is not your fault that the employee chose to display unacceptable behaviors—that was a choice he or she made. Therefore, do not apologize to them—you did nothing wrong.

- Your ability to hold staff accountable to their job affects the quality of the resident care that they deliver.

The performance review process is an opportunity for the manager and employee to meet in a nondistracting environment to share their perspectives on delivering resident care. If you remember to give just the facts, you will be heading in a successful direction with your evaluation process. Sometimes managers feel they have to pave the way for bad news or add a compliment when, in fact, the employee just wants to get down to business. In preparation for the meeting, the manager should have the following on their desk and readily available:

- Employee handbook with pages/sections marked that align with any discussion related to unacceptable behaviors

- Any policies/procedures you need to address with the employee

- Letters or phone calls of praise from coworkers, visitors, residents, etc.

- Their current job description

- Achievements, such as certifications for specialties or clinical skills

- Recognition related to a community project (e.g., Special Olympics, the local PTA)

- Copies of any electronic communications to validate concerns, such as inappropriate use of clock in/out or inappropriate use of Internet or facility e-mail communications

- Details about committee involvement

- Attendance records and documentation of participation at departmental meetings

- Copies of any regulation that the employee is not following (e.g., hand washing guidelines from the Joint Commission, Occupational Safety and Health Administration requirements on the use of protective equipment, etc.)

- Information from any patient charts that will be discussed (e.g., an ongoing documentation concern that is being reviewed)

- Salary information, if approved by human resources in advance

- Copy of previous year's evaluation tool to use for comparison or reference

Preparing the environment

Once you are prepared mentally and have all of your documents in order, the next step is to prepare the environment for the meeting. Employees have a right to privacy and confidentiality during their evaluations, and it is important for you to send the message that you respect that right. Here are some tips on preparing the environment for an evaluation:

- Give your pager to another manager to respond to calls during the evaluation time

- Hang a note on the door of your office that simply states, "Meeting in progress. Please do not disturb."

- Inform the operator that you will not be available for the next hour, and ask him or her not to overhead page you but instead to direct your calls to_____.

- Program your phone to ring once and then go directly to voice mail, or shut the ringer off.

- Arrange your office so that the desk does not separate you and the employee. The best scenario is to have two chairs without a desk between them. However, have the desk near your chair so you can easily access any documents needed during the discussion.

Preparing the employee

The employee needs to have some responsibility in the evaluation process; the meeting is for them, after all. Therefore, to encourage the employee's involvement and responsibility, the manager should send a memo to him or her at least two weeks prior to the date of the scheduled performance review, informing the employee of its date, time, and location. Make the memo a positive experience for the employee by using key phrases such as "opportunity for their input" or "looking forward to helping them reach their goals for the next year." Request that the employee arrive prepared to discuss:

- Recommendations for their job description

- Suggestions for improvement of resident care

- Any letters, achievements, etc., they would like to add to the review

- Their short- and long-term goals (professional or personal)

(If your department uses peer reviews as part of the evaluation process, and it is the employee's responsibility to ensure that peers have completed the forms, remind the employee of this fact as well.)

You probably know the personalities of staff that report to you better than anyone in the organization. This knowledge is the key to an effective evaluation. Some staff will need more prodding when asked about topics such as goal setting, and others will come to the meeting with their goals typed. Some staff will not prepare at all for the evaluation—in this case, remember that it is not your responsibility to do the preparation and collection of information; it's theirs.

You know which staff members excel in areas of customer service, exceed minimal clinical requirements, get involved as preceptors for new hires, and so on. Dedicating time to think about your staff's personalities and being prepared for the possibility of their responses allows you time to consider beforehand your options for response. Also, use this information to prepare yourself with methods of recognition/reward that align with the personality of the individual.

Setting goals

Managers and staff typically have approached goals as items to fill in on an evaluation tool or as important only for people who have not performed to the level of expectation set by the organization. In reality, however, goals are important not only for the employee but also for the manager. Well-developed goals clarify for both parties:

- Specific actions and behaviors the employee is expected to demonstrate

- Deadlines the employee has been given to accomplish certain achievements

Although it is important that some of the goals directly relate to the role and job description of the employee, the manager should also consider looking beyond the walls of the building in which the employee works. Part of the role of a manager is to help staff identify a long-term vision for themselves as well as to incorporate and support, when possible, goals outside of the organization.

Managers should not let their fear of losing good staff get in the way of encouraging and motivating people to advance their skills or improve themselves. Even though several years down the road you may no longer have those employees in the department, you must factor in what they brought to the team while they were advancing and working with your department:

- Positive attitude

- Ongoing advanced skills and knowledge that they shared with others

- Motivation to learn new techniques and skills

Some goal setting will not be as positive, such as setting goals related to punctuality or attendance. In these types of scenarios, it is vital that the manager be very specific and clear about what they expect of the employee:

- "The goal is that in the next 14 days there will be no reports of your tardiness. Do you have any questions about this that I can answer for you?"

- "The goal we have agreed on today is that you will attend and participate in the next department meeting."

For goals to be effective, the manager should ensure that they are:

- Observable

- Measurable

- Specific

- Realistic

- Given a time frame

Be cautious as you approach discussion of goals with staff members, and realize that your expectations of them may be unrealistic. Each individual has limitations on workload, ability to handle increased responsibilities, and feelings related to disappointment in the eyes of his or her manager. By agreeing on goals together, you minimize the opportunity of making the performance evaluation a time employees fear rather than one to which they look forward.

Communication tools

The evaluation is a perfect opportunity for the manager to show staff that their input is valued and their ideas are needed to continue improving resident care processes. Prepare one or two key questions that you can offer to each staff member that will prompt a response that involves an employee action, such as the following:

- If you could change one thing about the department, what would it be?

- Is there anything in particular that you have accomplished over the past year that I may not be aware of that you would like to share with me?

- You are such an asset to this department. What is it that motivates you to come to work every day?

- Where do you see the department heading with all of the legislative changes pending that we discussed at our staff meeting last week?

- How do you think we can better prepare ourselves to meet the increase in census we are having?

- What can I or the organization do to help you do your job better?

The keys to an effective performance evaluation process

The value of a performance evaluation is measured in its effectiveness. An effective evaluation process is organized and consistent and requires that you:

- Have a designated schedule for the year that identifies whose evaluation is due, when their reminder letter should be sent, and the actual date of the review

- Have a process by which the manager can note/log:

  - Ongoing positive performances and areas that need improvement or are unacceptable

  - Dates/times of the above scenarios

      – Feedback from peers, patients, etc.

      – Newspaper stories and other information on achievements of staff outside of the organization

- Hold the employee accountable for gathering some of the material/data required

- Prepare yourself and the environment

- Establish a process that follows up on short-term goals and ensures employee compliance

- Ensure that time is spent with staff throughout the year, both formally and informally, to discuss or address their performance

Case Study: An evaluation that sparks anger

Q Naomi becomes upset during her evaluation after you inform her that her raise will be affected by 2% because she does not have the material required for the evaluation, such as copies of letters and documentation that she completed the required educational components. She uses an angry tone, and she is having difficulty moving on to the next section of the evaluation: her goals. How do you move Naomi from her place of anger and redirect her attention so you can complete the evaluation process?

A *The most important issue is Naomi's inappropriate behavior: her angry tone. First, clarify your expectations. Say, "Naomi, I understand that you are angry because of the effect on your salary increase; however, you were aware of the requirements prior to today's meeting. As we continue and complete the performance review, I expect to be treated more respectfully. If you feel that you cannot complete this evaluation today, please let me know and I would be happy to reschedule it."*

Pause and allow her time to think about her options. Continue, "Understand that noncompletion of your performance review will result in disciplinary action, and I do not want to see that happen. Let's work together now and use this time as an opportunity to complete your evaluation and to find a way to schedule you for those education requirements."

Recommended reading

1. Guyant, Al, et al. *Manager's Tough Questions Answer Book.* New Jersey: Prentice Hall, 1996.

2. Nelson, Bob. *1001 Ways to Energize Employees.* New York: Workman Publishing, 1997.

3. Nelson, Bob. *1001 Ways to Reward Employees.* New York: Workman Publishing, 1994.

4. Deck, Michele, L. *Instant Teaching Tools for Health Care Educators.* St. Louis: Mosby, 1995.

5. Tamblyn, Doni, et al. *The Big Book of Humorous Training Games.* New York: McGraw-Hill, 2000.

6. Wright, Donna. *The Ultimate Guide to Competency Assessment in Healthcare.* Minneapolis: PESI Healthcare, 1998.

CHAPTER 11

Standards of care

A profession is an occupation or career, such as law, medicine, or engineering that requires advanced educational preparation and specialized study. A professional is an individual who is engaged in certain careers, such as lawyers, doctors, and nurses. Professionals are educated and qualified, and often must pass a licensure exam, pay a fee, and be licensed to perform these duties. Most professions change regularly due to new research, technology, and other information. Continuing education is necessary to maintain the professionals' knowledge and learn new trends and standards of practice. In some states and professions, continuing education is mandatory to maintain licensure. However, it is usually necessary, even if it is optional in your state. Professional behavior involves assuming responsibility and conforming to the standards of the profession. A professional may be considered a skilled practitioner or expert.

Professional responsibility

Professional responsibility is assuming responsibility for your own actions, abiding by the law, knowing and applying current standards of practice, and keeping the residents' best interests primary. "Professional responsibility is a paradigm case of the moral responsibility that arises from the special knowledge that one possesses. It is mastery of a special body of advanced knowledge, particularly knowledge which bears directly on the well-being of others that demarcates a profession. As custodians of special knowledge which bears on human well-being, professionals are constrained by special moral responsibilities; that is, moral requirements to apply their knowledge in ways that benefit the rest of the society."[1]

Adhering to professional standards of practice or standards of care protects the residents from injury. This protects both the professional and healthcare facility from liability. Because of ongoing changes and new information, this is an area in which your knowledge must constantly be updated. One important professional responsibility is to do what is necessary to maintain knowledge of professional standards of practice and proficiency in the necessary skills. For example, a resident who is a full code goes into cardiac arrest. None of the nurses on duty has a current CPR card. Should you start CPR or wait for EMS? Neither choice is a good one. Your employer is not responsible for keeping your CPR card current, although they likely will be sanctioned if you fail to fulfill your professional responsibility in maintaining your certificate.

CPR is a skill you need to meet the standards of care for the residents for whom you are responsible. A long-term care facility must provide services in compliance with accepted professional practices and standards. As part of the nurses' professional responsibility:

- The nurse assumes responsibility and accountability for individual nursing judgment and actions.[3]

- The nurse promotes, advocates for, and strives to protect the health, safety, and rights of the residents.[4]

- The nurse exercises informed judgment and uses individual competence and qualifications as criteria in seeking consultation, accepting responsibilities, and delegating nursing activities to others. The nurse collaborates with members of the health professions to meet the health needs of the public.[5]

- The nurse is responsible and accountable for individual nursing practice and determines the appropriate delegation of tasks consistent with the nurse's obligation to provide optimum resident care.[6]

Adhering to professional standards

All professions have standards and practices for their members. The standard of care is the degree of care or competence that one is expected to exercise in a particular circumstance or role.[7] In the nursing profession, the American Nurses Association (ANA), professional organizations, and state licensure boards identify standards for nurses to follow. Failure to provide care that meets or exceeds these standards may cause resident harm and is cause for disciplinary action against the licensee.

The old adage "Ignorance of the law is no excuse" can be applied to professional standards. Ignorance of professional standards is no excuse, either. Nurses must become familiar with the standards for their area of practice. You do not have to join a professional organization to learn and apply the standards. You will be held accountable to the standards of professional organizations, such as the ANA, even if you are not a member.

The standard of care is what a reasonable, prudent professional would do based on his or her education, experience, institutional policies and procedures, standards set by their professional organization(s), textbooks, research, and professional literature. Remember that many individual standards apply to the care of each resident. The standard of care is not what the best professional would do, but rather what any reasonable professional would do in the same or similar circumstances.

Technology and practices change rapidly, and professionals must remain current and keep up with these changes. Facilities must strive to keep their policies and procedures up-to-date. If the facility policies and procedures are outdated, research and evidence-based practices will supersede them if a lawsuit is filed. For example, in the early 1990s, government research indicated that nurses should not massage red areas to stimulate circulation.[8] Prior to this, massaging was an age-old method of pressure ulcer prevention. A nurse documents that he or she vigorously massaged a red area daily, according to facility policy. If the area subsequently ulcerates, the evidence-based government research and information supersede the outdated practice of massaging. The nurse and facility may be found liable for contributing to pressure ulcer development.

If a professional holds certifications and advanced education, he or she is held to the same standard as other professional individuals with like qualifications. For example, if a registered nurse holds a certification in gerontologic nursing care, he or she is held to a higher standard than nurses without this certification.

The long-term care facility laws are quite clear regarding the applicable standards of care:

- §483.20(k)(3) The services provided or arranged by the facility must (I) Meet professional standards of quality and; §483.20(k)(3)(ii) Be provided by qualified persons in accordance with each resident's written plan of care.

- Interpretive Guidelines §483.20(k)(3)(i) "Professional standards of quality" means services that are provided according to accepted standards of clinical practice. Standards may apply to care provided by a particular clinical discipline or in a specific clinical situation or setting. Standards regarding quality care practices may be published by a professional organization, licensing board, accreditation body or other regulatory agency. Recommended practices to achieve desired resident outcomes may also be found in clinical literature.[9]

Protocols and routine practices

Some facilities have a set of protocols or standards used in the care of all residents. Because these are routine practices, they are usually not listed on the care plans. The care plans list only additions and exceptions to the usual routines. (How care plans are managed is a facility determination.) If your facility decides to implement protocols and standards for routine resident care, avoid writing the standards yourself. Involve appropriate staff, including residents and nursing assistants (and others) where appropriate, in the development and adoption of standards and protocols that affect overall resident care. Staff are much more likely to make this type of system successful if they have ownership in protocol development.

An experienced medical/legal reviewer can easily identify the various components of the nursing process during a medical record review. Years ago, nurses neglected documentation when they were busy, focusing instead on resident care. "Put the patient ahead of the paper" was a common expression. Today, management must support nurses in finding a way to do both. Documentation is part of the resident's care, and nurses no longer have the luxury of choosing between providing care and keeping records.[10] Documentation validates that care was given. Sometimes, it proves that the facility was providing care it was paid to provide. It proves that standards of care were met. Documentation is an essential element of communication. Accurate and complete documentation is essential so others can determine what has been done. All healthcare practitioners rely on having accurate and thorough data on the medical record when they are completing their individual assessments and planning future clinical approaches to resident care.

Healthcare professionals have a broad knowledge of many subjects.

We have additional, specific, specialized knowledge in our selected areas of expertise and practice. Nevertheless, knowing all we need to know about every subject is impossible. For the most part, our generalized knowledge sustains us, but sometimes the nurse must learn more about applicable, current standards in subjects outside the specialty area. At the very least, professionals must familiarize themselves with the actions, uses, side effects, indications, contraindications, and precautions for new drugs. Aside from that, you may be faced with situations in which you will need to research standards, even if you think you know them cold.

Some of the simplest standards may be the most difficult to find, and you may need to be resourceful to find what you need. Published standards of practice come from many different sources. The Internet has become another important source. Thousands of standards can be accessed online, quickly and painlessly. Knowing and following the standards of practice for your profession and employment setting will ensure that residents receive quality care. Applying professional practice standards:

- Protects resident (and employee) safety

- Achieves desirable resident (care) outcomes

- Facilitates access to appropriate services and levels of healthcare

- Identifies the scope of accountability for nursing care

- Reduces nurse and facility liability and legal exposure

Quality of care

The Director of Nursing (DON) in long-term care maintains a constant vigil to assure that the physical, mental, and social needs of the residents are met. The DON develops systems for appropriate staffing, appropriate medical supervision, and appropriate therapeutic attention.[11]

Each resident must receive, and the facility must provide, the necessary care and services to attain or maintain the highest practicable physical, mental, and psychosocial well-being, in accordance with the comprehensive assessment and plan of care. Highest practicable is defined as the highest level of functioning and well-being possible, limited only by the individual's presenting functional status and potential for improvement or reduced rate of functional decline. Highest practicable is determined through the comprehensive interdisciplinary resident assessment, and by competently and thoroughly addressing the physical, mental, or psychosocial needs of the individual.

The facility must ensure that the resident obtains optimal improvement or does not deteriorate within the limits of the right to refuse treatment, and within the limits of recognized pathology and the normal aging process.[12] When a resident shows signs of decline, surveyors will review the record to determine whether the decline is unavoidable. A physician statement that the decline is unavoidable will be considered, but is not accepted at face value without a detailed investigation of the situation.

An accurate determination of unavoidable decline or failure to reach the highest practicable well-being may be made only if all of the following are present:

- An accurate and complete assessment

- An assessment-based care plan that has been consistently implemented

- The resident's response to care has been evaluated, and the care plan revised as necessary

Nursing process breakdown

The DON in long-term care advocates for the assessment and evaluation of outcomes in the long-term care facility and develops implementation strategies for negative outcomes.[13]

The medical model of operations (care) is designed to promote staff efficiency and provide for the residents' medical needs. Under the medical model, mealtimes usually dictate daily schedules and routines. Care may be driven by the third-party payers. Residents are not always involved in making the decisions affecting their care. Many facilities are finding that for holistic care, wellness, and optimal quality of life, care must reflect an integration of various models of care, including the medical model, the holistic, resident-centered model, the participatory model, and the wellness model of care.

When the nursing process breaks down in long-term care, it is usually due to one or more of the following:

- Lack of functional understanding of the nursing process itself

- Lack of understanding of the Omnibus Budget Reconciliation Act regulations

- Inability to differentiate between the medical model of care and holistic, resident-centered care

- Feeling stressed, overwhelmed, and spread too thin

Nurses must deliver competent care as demonstrated by the nursing process, including assessment, diagnosis, outcome identification, planning, implementation, and evaluation. The nursing process encompasses all significant actions taken by nurses in providing care to all clients, and forms the foundation of clinical decision-making.[14]

Frequently, the nursing process breaks down in the assessment stage. Occasionally, assessment is not done at all. More commonly, the resident is assessed, but personnel fail to act on the results of the assessment by calling the physician, providing continued reassessment, or taking whatever other actions are necessary. Sometimes assessment is not timely. The resident may have been deteriorating slowly for several days, but he or she is not assessed and physician notifications are not made until the situation is emergent or the resident unstable. Remember, once data have been collected, the nurse and facility are responsible for the information. Use the clinical assessment data and medical record information to take appropriate action based on your appraisal and evaluation of that data. When you collect data, you are obligated to use it.

Care planning

When making clinical judgments, nurses must base their decisions on consideration of consequences, which prescribe and justify nursing actions. The recipients of professional nursing services are entitled to high-quality nursing care.[15] The gerontological nurse collects data through assessment, analyzes the data, plans nursing care, implements the Plan, and evaluates the effectiveness of the Plan of Care. The process is fluid and ongoing to ensure quality nursing care. The gerontological nurse systematically evaluates the quality of care and effectiveness of nursing practice. The gerontological nurse considers factors related to safety and effectiveness in planning and delivering client care.[16]

Another area in which nursing process breakdown commonly occurs is care planning. This is usually because many nurses have mental blocks against care plans stemming from bad experiences in nursing school. Some nurses subscribe to the myth that the care plan is a means of paper compliance only, and is not an essential document in the care of the residents. Additionally, there are many fallacies about how care plans are to be structured and the format for identifying problems and needs. In truth, the facility is required to develop a comprehensive care plan, but there are no requirements for a prescribed format. Many facilities use the medical model of care to construct their care plans. This seems somewhat incongruent in a homelike environment. It also results in the "problem-need" format. It does not identify or use resident strengths to overcome needs.

The care plan cannot be separated from the nursing process. Facilities that keep the care plan in front of staff, update it as often as necessary, and use the plan as a tool for directing all resident care activities seldom deliver bad or dysfunctional care. Successful managers really do make this happen, and it shows in the quality of care delivered by the entire healthcare team. The care plan is probably the single most important document on your chart. It is much more than paper compliance. In fact, keeping the care plan on the chart limits its utility and accessibility. Using a Kardex format is often much more useful.

The probes for §483.20(k)(1) (the care planning rules) ask the following questions. As you can see, these are all issues discussed in your book as being important in reducing the risk of legal exposure:

- Does the care plan address the needs, strengths, and preferences identified in the comprehensive resident assessment?

- Is the care plan oriented toward preventing avoidable declines in functioning or functional levels? How does the care plan attempt to manage risk factors? Does the care plan build on resident strengths?

- Does the care plan reflect standards of current professional practice?

- Do treatment objectives have measurable outcomes?

- Corroborate information regarding the resident's goals and wishes for treatment in the plan of care by interviewing residents, especially those identified as refusing treatment.

- Determine whether the facility has provided adequate information to the resident so that the resident was able to make an informed choice regarding treatment.

- If the resident has refused treatment, does the care plan reflect the facility's efforts to find alternative means to address the problem?

Converting the system from one in which the care plan is considered paper compliance to one in which the care plan is a dynamic document requires considerable managerial time and effort. It also takes staff commitment. Without this commitment, the results may be abysmal. Staff resistance to change is a normal human phenomenon, but this document often evokes such strong feelings that some staff members may do all they can to actively resist change. Using the care plan is a worthwhile endeavor, and will make a difference in quality of care, quality of life, and reduced legal exposure.

To be viable, the care plan must be initiated on admission. All assessments will not be complete, but your preliminary plan should identify any obvious problems, risk factors, or conditions for which the resident was hospitalized. At this point, no one expects the plan to be perfect. It should be functional and should direct initial care until you know the resident better. Add to the plan as new information becomes available. The residents' conditions are not static. Changes in condition, problems, needs, strengths, and approaches must be added to the plan as often as necessary to ensure the plan is kept current. Like our residents, the plan evolves and changes. Care planning considerations include:

- The services provided or arranged by the facility must meet professional standards of quality. There should be evidence of assessment and care planning sufficient to meet the needs of newly admitted residents, prior to completion of the first comprehensive assessment and comprehensive care plan.[17]

- Facilities are responsible for assessing areas that are relevant to residents regardless of whether these areas are included in the Resident Assessment Instrument (RAI; The RAI is the minimum assessment tool, not the only assessment tool.[18]

- The care plan is a dynamic document that needs to be continually evaluated and appropriately modified based on measurable outcomes. This continual evaluation takes into consideration resident change relative to the initial baseline—in other words, if the resident has declined, stayed the same, or improved at a lesser rate than expected, then a modification in the care plan may be necessary.[19]

- As the process of problem identification is integrated with sound clinical interventions, the care plan becomes each resident's unique path toward achieving or maintaining his or her highest practicable level of well-being.[20]

- When the care plan is implemented in accordance with the standards of good clinical practice, then the care plan becomes powerful and practical, and represents the best approach to providing for the quality-of-care and quality-of-life needs of an individual resident.[21]

Developing an initial plan and updating the care plan are particularly problematic for long-term care facilities, which (technically) have up to 21 days to develop a comprehensive plan of care. A lot can happen in the first 21 days. In fact, this period is when the resident's risk factors may be greatest, because they are unfamiliar to staff. The resident is not familiar with the facility. During the first 21 days, safety risks, weight loss, inadequate fluid intake, and risk of skin breakdown can be particularly problematic.

Leaving the vulnerable resident without a plan for a prolonged period exposes him or her to serious hazards, and exposes the facility and its staff to the potential for liability. Having an interim plan that is imperfect (and not comprehensive) is certainly better than no plan at all. Using this plan is a key to successful care. Having a perfect piece of paper doesn't translate into excellent care, but you can make this happen. Use the plan for developing assignments and giving reports. Keep it in front of the staff. Update the plan promptly if the problems, goals, or approaches change, even if changes seem minor. Avoid discouraging unit staff from making changes to the plan. It is their plan for the resident's care. In some facilities, only the MDS nurse can change the plan. Facilities are encouraged to rethink this strategy. The MDS nurse most probably does not know of changes immediately after they occur, and is probably not on duty during the second and third shifts. Staff nurses and charge nurses are in a much better position to change and develop the plan.

After the Minimum Data Set (MDS) is done and the comprehensive long-term care plan is developed, the natural tendency is to bury the plan in the chart and not look at it until it is time for quarterly review. Although residents in this setting are more stable than those in acute care, the plan must be updated for changes in condition or it will be ineffective and inaccurate for directing care. Even stable residents are likely to require minor care plan changes during the three-month period between quarterly care plan reviews.

Used correctly, the plan evolves throughout the individual's stay in the facility. Information should be added or removed as often as necessary. If a change involves a single department, that department may make the change and implement the plan. If a change involves two or more departments, you may wish to bring the plan into care conference for a quick review and update. For example, the nurse nicks the skin slightly when clipping a resident's fingernails. This information should be added to the plan by the nurse on duty, because care for the cut is given only by the nursing department.

However, if the resident experiences an unplanned, undesirable weight loss, the nurse who identifies the loss should add the information to the plan of care. He or she should flag the plan for update at the next available care conference, because dietary, activities, and social services may also have responsibilities for managing the resident's weight loss. Whether you invite the resident and family to this update conference is a facility decision. Many facilities handle updates at the end of each regular care conference, with only staff members in attendance. Since updating the plan normally involves only minor changes, outside parties are usually not invited. However, they should be advised of the need for a change in the plan, and their suggestions (if any) included.

Additional care plan considerations

Although the MDS drives the long-term care facility comprehensive plan, consider all other assessments, as well as other contents of the medical record when developing the plan. List any potential risk factor, medication, treatment, or other order that modifies or increases a risk factor or requires special monitoring. For example, a nursing assessment or MDS may not identify problems related to medication interactions or side effects. A review of the physician's orders or medication record will identify potential problems in this area. Drugs such as anticoagulants interact with many other foods and drugs, and almost always increase the resident's risk of adverse outcomes. Because of this risk, the drugs and special monitoring should be listed on the care plan. Use your professional judgment to ensure this information is added to the plan. Avoid assuming that all other caregivers know what you know. They probably don't. Write it down!

Most nursing boards have rules that require nursing diagnoses to be the basis of the care plan. Nursing assistants and other paraprofessional workers usually do not understand nursing diagnoses terminology. If you list nursing diagnoses on the care plans to comply with the requirements of the state nurse practice act, you may wish to write a simple problem in parentheses next to it. For example, if a resident has a nursing diagnosis such as "deficit fluid volume" or "risk for deficient fluid volume," you may wish to write "dehydration" or "risk for dehydration" or "inadequate fluid intake" next to it so all caregivers understand the problem. Consider the care plan location.

In many states, the long-term care rules require facilities to make the plans available to all direct-care staff. Burying the plan in a medical record with hundreds of other documents makes it inaccessible, and staff will be less likely to sift through the charts each shift to review the care plans. In some facilities, nursing assistant staff are not permitted to read the charts. This is somewhat incongruous if the chart contains the only copy of the plans of care! Some facilities have had problems with care plans disappearing. Sadly, this is usually done in retaliation for perceived managerial injustices, because staff know that developing new care plans requires a great investment in management time and effort. Copying the care plans after care conference is a simple task. Store the copies in an office or secure medical records file. Although the copies are not updated when changes occur, they are a good starting point if you must rewrite an entire plan. For day-to-day unit operations, using a notebook or Kardex for care plans may be a more useful approach.

Some facilities make copies of the care plan and store them in notebooks with flow sheets, according to team assignments. The original plans are maintained in the medical record. Consider the options that work best for your facility, but do all you can to ensure the plans are accessible to, and used by, floor-level staff.

Care plan checklist

The care plan should be:

- Created upon admission, listing potential safety problems, high-risk conditions, and obvious medical and psychosocial problems.

    - Use common sense when developing admission problems. If the resident fell at home, list him or her as being at risk for falls. If he or she has an indwelling catheter, list the potential for catheter infection. Formal written assessments are not needed to identify these potential admission risks. The problem can be removed later if it does not pertain to the resident's current needs.

- Further developed and refined after the MDS and other admission assessments have been completed.

- Interdisciplinary.

- Individualized to the residents' unique problems, needs, and risk factors.

- Reflective of the residents' strengths.

- Reflective of the care being given.

- Updated as often as necessary to ensure the plan is current.

- Readily and freely available to direct caregiving staff.

- Used as the basis for making assignments and giving report to staff.

- Reviewed each shift with direct-care personnel (problems, goals, approaches).

- Implemented consistently by all staff (problems, goals, approaches).

- Regularly evaluated (effectiveness of problems, goals, approaches).

- Revised if approaches are ineffective, inappropriate, or no longer relevant, or if new problems develop.

Documentation should reflect observations, care given and resident response, and evaluation of care listed in the plan. Consistent, individualized care is crucial to positive resident outcomes and safety. Documentation in one area of the medical record should be consistent with other areas of the record. Take care to ensure information is not contradictory. Make sure care is in keeping with the full plan. For example, physical therapy is working with a confused resident and determines he can safely ambulate independently for short distances, such as with a walker in his room.

Nursing documentation should not state, "restrained in chair at all times for safety." This defeats the purpose of the therapy, and probably contradicts the therapists' professional judgment and physician orders. Additionally, you are being paid to provide therapy and supervise the resident's ambulation in his or her room. A managed care payer source may deny payment for the entire month because the care was not delivered as ordered, and according to the prescribed and approved plan of care.

The care plan keeps everyone apprised of the resident's strengths, problems, and needs. Your commitment to developing and using the plan is a key to success. Changing the system and making it care plan–driven takes time and effort. However, over the long term, it saves time and energy. Most important, it ensures resident safety, improves satisfaction, enhances the quality of care, and improves quality of life in your facility.

Quality of life

The Director of Nursing in long-term care continuously seeks out those indicators which will define quality of life in the long-term care facility and monitors or develops tools which will monitor those indicators. The DON seeks collaboration with other disciplines in the development and monitoring of such indicators.[22]

Along with the quality of medical care residents receive, the quality of each individual's life is an important way to measure the success of a facility's caregiving. Quality of life is the state of being that results from the reconciliation of one's abilities and resources with one's collection of perceptions and beliefs that define meaning and purpose for life. Remember personal indicators as well as medical ones when measuring quality of life. Ask residents and family members how they measure the quality of care, quality of life, and customer satisfaction.[23]

Making a distinction between quality of clinical care and quality of life is appropriate, because these aspects of facility care are monitored and assessed very differently. Quality of care is quantitative, whereas quality of life is qualitative. Measurement of clinical care tends to be a matter of objective observation and examination of the person and comparison of that person's data to an established clinical standard of practice. Quality of life, on the other hand, depends on the subjective view of each individual, a far more difficult thing to measure. Two residents could receive comparable clinical care, yet one resident views his quality of life as good, and the other rates his quality of life as poor.

Projects such as participating in pet and music therapy, environmental and art enhancement, and multigenerational activities involving local elementary school children, are things that enhance the quality of many residents' lives. Interpersonal interventions that reduce learned helplessness and restore the residents' sense of autonomy and control also enhance quality of life. Residents who believe they are receiving good quality of care, and those who are satisfied with the quality of their lives, are not likely to complain to the state or file a lawsuit. In fact, they are apt to praise and defend the facility when questioned by surveyors.

Cultural change in long-term care

The Eden Alternative®, Pioneer®, and other culture-changing programs have been very successful because they view aging as a distinct stage of human development. The medical model of care reinforces the defeatist attitude that declines are not optional in aging and that we must learn to live with the deterioration. According to the medical model, the greatest problems facility residents face are disease, disability, and decline. Undoubtedly, many declines accompany the aging process, but the human spirit can and does continue to grow.

The culture-change movement approaches care for all residents, including those with dementia, with the attitude that everyone has the capacity for continued personal growth if provided an environment that supports and nurtures that growth. Eden is based on the belief that the major problems of aging are loneliness, helplessness, and boredom, which cause a disintegration of the residents' spirit.

Many of the principles are based on an ethical framework and broad thinking about social responsibility, ecology, and anthropology. They promote autonomy and control over the everyday matters in residents' lives, noting that some residents thrive when given small challenges, such as making food choices or tending a plant. Eden and other alternative movements promote the philosophy that the focus of long-term care should be on "care" rather than on the notions of "treatment" or "therapy" inherent in a medical model. Whether you agree or disagree with this philosophy, it is evident that many elderly individuals thrive in this type of environment, and the quality of their lives appears to be excellent. Borrowing successful ideas from the culture-change movement and implementing them in your facility may be very beneficial to the residents.

Determining whether life is worth living is a highly subjective and personal viewpoint, particularly when an individual is faced with physical or mental impairment and protracted dependency and institutionalization. The current long-term care laws are based on an activist vision that includes the reduction or elimination of restraints; therapeutic activities using music, art, pets, plants, and intergenerational exchanges; architectural and design alterations that enhance safety and autonomy; an emphasis on rehabilitation and discharge,[2] and other options. Assisted living has become a very popular option for higher functioning individuals. These things all promote the philosophy that life is worth living.

Many facilities do not have the means or desire to change their philosophy or culture of care. Suggestions for enhancing quality of life in the traditional long-term care facility are:

- Providing choices, such as:

  - When to get up

  - When does the resident want to eat and drink

  - What does he or she want to eat and drink

  - When does the resident want to bathe or shower

- Facility response to resident needs:

  - Flexible staffing schedules

  - Cooperation among staff

  - Everyone pitches in; cross-training

  - Assigning a staff person to advocate for each resident's wants and needs

  - Providing support

- Additional suggestions:

  - Teach staff about aging and increase their capacity to understand individual residents' perspectives

  - Promote and enable a normalization of social relationships

  - Recognize how aging affects things such as diet, identity, and relationships

  - Treat each resident as an individual; avoid stereotyping

  - Provide continuity of care through use of the care plan

  - Treat residents as your equals; work with them toward a common goal

The relationship between the nurse manager and paraprofessional caregivers is also believed to affect the quality of residents' lives. Residents do well in an environment in which the supervisor and paraprofessional have developed skill in:

- Empathy

- Reliability

Resident quality of life is also enhanced when facility staff:

- Nurture personal relationships with the residents

- Know residents' needs and assign fair workloads

- Mentor other staff

- Can delegate

- Can turn to the Administrator for advice

- Communicate well and share information

- Eliminate obstacles that prevent supervisors from doing their work

Residents with dementia

In years past, providing reality orientation (RO) was a very popular care plan intervention. Most facilities have "RO Boards" that are changed daily, and list information such as the day and date, season, weather, and holiday facts, when appropriate. Although the daily bulletin boards are helpful, formal reality orientation is often unsuccessful and may upset some residents.

Staff must learn to relate to cognitively impaired residents' reality, instead of imposing their reality on the residents. For example, if the resident worries that the children need to be fed, reassure her that someone has taken care of that. Or ask the resident about what she likes to cook and how she prepares it. Doing this restores the state of mind she is seeking, reducing her anxiety. These are not lies. It is true that someone has tended to things the resident is worried about, although the issue is probably no longer relevant.

Restoring the resident's state of mind is an excellent way of relieving agitation. Understanding our reality is not a realistic goal for most residents with dementia. Entering into their reality is a therapeutic measure that improves and enhances quality of life!

References

1. Nightingale F. (1859). Notes on nursing. London: Harrison and Sons, 1859, p. 74

2. Mann M. (2000). Research ethics glossary. University of Nebraska. Online. www.unmc.edu/ethics/words.html. Accessed 11/13/05.

3. American Nurses Association (Eds). (2002). Code for Nurses with Interpretive Statements. Washington, D.C. American Nurses Publishing.

4. American Nurses Association (Eds.). (2002). Code for Nurses with Interpretive Statements. Washington, D.C. American Nurses Publishing.

5. American Nurses Association (Eds.). (2002). Code for Nurses with Interpretive Statements. Washington, D.C. American Nurses Publishing.

6. American Nurses Association (Eds). (2002). Code for Nurses with Interpretive Statements. Washington, D.C. American Nurses Publishing.

7. Merriam-Webster's dictionary of law (1996). Merriam-Webster's, Incorporated.

8. U.S. Department of Health and Human Services (Eds). (1992). Pressure Ulcers in Adults: Prediction and Prevention. Rockville, MD. Agency for Health Care Policy and Research.

9. Centers for Medicare & Medicaid Services. (2004). State Operations Manual.

10. Richards, M. (2001). Documentation - a vital and essential element of the nursing process. Survey Savvy. Des Moines, Briggs Corporation.

11. National Association of Directors of Nursing Administration/Long Term Care (NADONA) (eds). (2000). Standards of Practice (4th edition). Cincinnati, OH. National Association of Directors of Nursing Administration/Long Term Care.

12. §483.25 State Operations Manual Revision 8 (2005).

13. National Association of Directors of Nursing Administration/Long Term Care (NADONA) (eds). (2000). Standards of Practice (4th edition). Cincinnati, OH. National Association of Directors of Nursing Administration/Long Term Care.

14. American Nurses Association. (1998). Standards of clinical nursing practice. Washington, D.C. American Nurses Publishing.

15. American Nurses Association (eds.). Code for Nurses. (2002). Washington, D.C. American Nurses Publishing.

16. American Nurses Association (eds). (1995). Scope and Standards of Gerontological Nursing Practice. Washington, D.C. American Nurses Publishing.

17. State Operations Manual. Probes for §483.20(k)(3)(i).

18. Morris, J.N., Murphy, K., Nonemaker, S. (1996). Long-term care facility resident assessment instrument (RAI) user's manual. Des Moines. Briggs Corp.

19. Morris, J.N., Murphy, K., Nonemaker, S. (1996). Long-term care facility resident assessment instrument (RAI) user's manual. Des Moines. Briggs Corp.

20. Morris, J.N., Murphy, K., Nonemaker, S. (1996). Long-term care facility resident assessment instrument (RAI) user's manual. Des Moines. Briggs Corp.

21. Morris, J.N., Murphy, K., Nonemaker, S. (1996). Long-term care facility resident assessment instrument (RAI) user's manual. Des Moines. Briggs Corp.

22. National Association of Directors of Nursing Administration/Long Term Care (NADONA) (eds). (2000). Standards of Practice (4th edition). Cincinnati, OH. National Association of Directors of Nursing Administration/Long Term Care.

23. Wisconsin Department of Health and Family Services. (2000). Care planning 2000 guideline. Madison. Bureau of Quality Assurance and Wisconsin Board on Aging and Long-term Care. Online. www.dhfs.wisconsin.gov/rl_DSL/Publications/ care2000.pdf. Accessed 3/15/04.

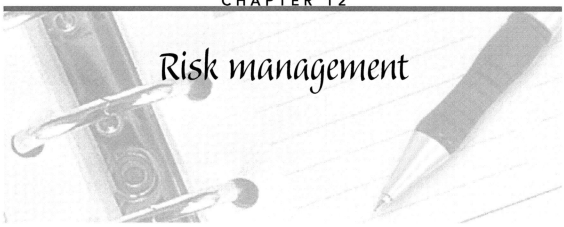

Risk management

Use of outside resources

If the facility does not employ a qualified professional person to furnish a specific service to be provided by the facility, the facility must have that service furnished to residents by a person or agency outside the facility under an arrangement described in section 1861(w) of the Act or an agreement described in paragraph (h)(2) of this section. Arrangements as described in section 1861(w) of the Act or agreements pertaining to services furnished by outside resources must specify in writing that the facility assumes responsibility for:

- Obtaining services that meet professional standards and principles that apply to professionals providing services in such a facility; and

- The timeliness of the services.[1]

Although 1861(w) is really not relevant to our purposes here, it is mentioned in the *Long-Term Care State Operations Manual* several times, where contracts are concerned. To satisfy your intellectual curiosity, it says:

"(w)(1) The term 'arrangements' is limited to arrangements under which receipt of payment by the hospital, critical access hospital, skilled nursing facility, home health agency, or hospice program (whether in its own right or as agent), with respect to services for which an individual is entitled to have payment made under this title, discharges the liability of such individual or any other person to pay for the services." It continues with (w)(2), which describes utilization review activities.

These services are needed (or potentially will be needed) by all residents. The facility is expected to have contracts (or letters of agreement) with an individual or company that provides these services to facility residents:

- Transfer agreement (hospital)

- Social services

- Dietitian

- Pharmacy/pharmacist

- Medical director

Facilities are required to provide certain services through their employees or by contracting for the services. For example, some facilities employ full-time dietitians and therapists. If they do not, they are expected to sign a contract (or letter of agreement) with an individual or company who provides these services to facility residents. Facilities are required to provide these services, if needed by the residents:

- Laboratory

- X-ray

- Therapy—physical (PT), occupational (OT), speech (ST), mental health/mental retardation (MHMR), respiratory (RT)

- Dentist

- Podiatrist

- Eye care

- Hearing

If the services are not provided in the facility, the facility is expected to assist the resident in locating the necessary service, and facilitating transportation through facility van, volunteers, family members, or another acceptable method.

Other contracts and agreements

Facilities may also have contracts with other providers, such as:

- Ambulance, medivan, or other form of nonemergency transportation

- Alternative housing, if evacuation of the facility is necessary

– Transportation to alternate housing, such as city bus or school bus

• Other suppliers, such as drinking water if the water supply is interrupted

The administrator will maintain many other miscellaneous contracts, such as pest control, elevator maintenance, fire extinguisher maintenance, oxygen supplier, dialysis center, hospice, and so forth. The nature and type of these agreements vary widely, and will not be discussed here.

Quality and timeliness of service

The federal requirements make facilities responsible for quality or timeliness of service, or both. Note that for lab and x-ray services, "the facility is responsible for the quality and timeliness of the services." This is important, because it is an area in which communication commonly breaks down.

If a lawsuit ensues, there is often a considerable amount of finger pointing between the facility and the outside provider regarding who is to blame. Most facilities have a contract with a lab or x-ray provider who comes to the facility. Having a method of tracking and ordering routine lab tests is essential. Once labs and x-ray have been done, there must be a system for ensuring reports are received in a timely manner, and that physician notifications and facility responses are timely.

Physician notification of abnormal values and nursing actions

Faxing a pile of normal and abnormal lab reports to the physician office may not constitute proper notification. In some situations, the facility continues to have the responsibility for identifying potential problems in the laboratory reports and notifying the physician by phone. This is especially true in coagulation tests and laboratory values suggesting dehydration, which are both commonly overlooked by nursing personnel.

A nurse must review the lab reports soon after they are returned to the facility and determine whether the values warrant phone notification or further nursing action. The tracking system should make it evident if lab reports have not been returned by the lab within a reasonable period of time. Nurses should be able to tell at a glance if they are missing, then contact the lab to resolve the problem.

Additionally, nurses are responsible for recognizing conditions and risk factors for which we have nursing diagnoses. For example, these are common nursing diagnoses:

• Risk for fluid volume imbalance

• Excess fluid volume

- Deficit fluid volume

- Risk for deficient fluid volume

These conditions are readily identified through abnormal laboratory values. Dehydration is one of the most common causes of hospitalization in the over-65 age group. The resident is often in critical condition with profound hypotension before the problem is identified and treated. All long-term care nurses must be able to identify laboratory values suggesting dehydration. Blood urea nitrogen (BUN) should be measured regularly in high-risk residents. Nurses must understand the meaning of abnormal BUN values and act on them. They must be able to identify signs of possible dehydration. The nurse finding an abnormal BUN must assess the resident. Fax the laboratory values to the physician, but follow up promptly by making phone contact. Discuss the assessment findings and significance of the lab values, and ask the physician for recommendations/orders. Values of concern that warrant nursing action include:

- BUN over 22 mg/dl.

- Elevated hematocrit (greater than three times the hemoglobin).

- Potassium below 3.5.

- Chloride over 107.

- Sodium over 147 (suggests severe dehydration).

- Elevated serum creatinine.

- A creatinine greater than 1.5 suggests renal disease. If elevated, determine the BUN/ Creatinine ratio. Divide the BUN by the creatinine. Values over 23 suggest dehydration.

If a resident experiences any of the values listed here, direct physician notification is necessary. In addition to orders for current care, request orders for follow-up monitoring after treatment. Request a physician order for routine laboratory monitoring in high-risk residents. Update the care plan. Notify the facility dietitian on his or her next visit. Consider adding intake and output monitoring to the care plan. Carefully evaluate the resident's daily fluid intake with his or her minimum fluid requirements. Write additional nursing orders on the care plan, and pass them on in your shift report. Document the notifications, actions taken, and resident response.

As you can see, nursing responsibility to the resident does not stop with faxing an abnormal report to the physician. Your responsibility for completing the nursing process continues, even if there are no new physician orders addressing the problem. Depending on the abnormal lab value, nursing responsibility may entail a minor care plan adjustment and nothing else. Rarely does an abnormal lab value require no action at all. Grasping and acting on this simple concept will prevent many resident complications and greatly reduce the potential for legal exposure. The facility is responsible for the resident's welfare, not just passing on information to the physician.

Risk management

Your facility will have a formal or informal risk-management program to reduce the risk of liability. Your insurance carrier probably has very specific policies and procedures for risk-management. They can also be an invaluable source of information on reducing legal exposure. Some facilities have a formal risk manager position, whereas others have a corporate risk management office. There are no "cookbook approaches" or "quick fixes" to guarantee successful risk management.

Following facility guidelines, policies, and procedures is always the best approach to take. Additionally, you and your personnel must be proactive, not reactive. Risk management and quality assurance are closely entwined. Ensuring the highest quality care for residents and protecting your facility from liability are constant concerns that parallel each other. In addition to following the formal risk-management program, some practical ways to reduce liability are:

- Make customer service your first priority. Make the residents feel important and appreciated.

- Provide consistency in caregivers and in the care given.

- Ensure that direct caregivers provide input into the plan of care. Some staff resent it when the plan is devised and dictated to them by department heads who do not know the resident well. The resident will benefit because these workers have in-depth knowledge of resident needs. Staff will feel empowered and will strive to make the plan work because they have ownership in it.

- Establish solid, trusting relationships with residents and families.

- Identify dissatisfied residents and family members. Address and resolve their concerns.

- Incorporate good communication and customer relations into your ongoing staff development program.

- Strive to maintain positive relationships and keep communication open with residents and responsible parties.

- Identify potential risk factors for all residents and address them with a preventive plan of care, which is updated as often as necessary.

- Anticipate and prevent adverse occurrences whenever possible.

- Provide thorough explanations of the care plan, taking time to answer questions. Identify residents who need extra services or support and provide it.

- Use skill, tact, and sensitivity when managing adverse events. Remain calm.

"The strategic planning process is not stagnant. In fact, it is fair to say that the plan is never complete. It changes continuously in order to maintain a strong presence in a complex environment. The plan becomes a blueprint and guide to move the unit, the department and/or the organization in a forward, focused and positive direction."[2]

- Document thoroughly and objectively.

- Make it a point to find out what your customers want, need, and value by asking them. In this situation, you will often get better information through regular informal meetings with residents, responsible parties, and staff than through formal meetings. Use active listening skills and compassion. Be responsive.

- Be a good employer. Make work fun for your staff. Be receptive to their suggestions.

- Ask your risk manager or legal counsel to review all contracts with outside parties.

- Verify the licensure status of all physicians, nurses, and others holding a professional license. Having a photocopy is not adequate. Check with the licensure board. You can do this online in many states. Likewise, check the nursing assistant registry. Follow state laws and facility policies for criminal history checks.

- Maintain current photographs of all residents. Keep these with the medication record, if possible. In any event, they should be accessible 24 hours a day.

- Keep a close eye on pressure ulcers by monitoring weekly; formally monitor them through the quality assurance program.

- Be familiar with, adhere to, and monitor standards of care. Make sure facility policies and practices reflect current standards.

- Your staff do not willfully break the law. Teach them the various laws and regulations governing long-term care, and describe how to comply with them.

- Monitor for, investigate, and analyze all incidents. Know what, how, and why they happened. Adjust care plans promptly to reduce the risk and prevent incidents from recurring.

- Study and learn from mistakes. Avoid blaming individuals. Analyze and correct systemic errors associated with increased risk and adverse outcomes.

- Develop, maintain, and promote a functional quality assurance committee. Committee members should include front-line workers. Stress the important of the quality assurance program.

Each insurer and underwriter is different, but to negotiate the most acceptable insurance premium, long-term care facilities should have policies, procedures, and effective programs for:

- Staffing issues, including:

  - Orientation and initial training

  - Employee background and criminal history checks

- Operations issues, including:

  - Medical records policies and retention practices

  - Privacy and security of medical records

  - Prompt reporting of potential occurrences

- Resident safety practices, including:

  - Fall prevention program

  - Restraint reduction program

  - Medication monitoring to reduce the risk of errors

  - Program for residents who wander and are at risk for elopement

  - Prevention of abuse, neglect, and misappropriation of property

- Resident care, including:

  - Pressure ulcer prevention program

  - Pain management policies and procedures

  - Effective program for monitoring residents and meeting nutrition and hydration needs

  - Hospice or program for holistic care of residents with known terminal illness

Abuse and neglect

Many lawsuits include complaints of resident abuse and neglect, which open a gigantic can of worms, including the possibility of criminal prosecution. However, preventing abuse and neglect is part of your risk-management program. You should also provide ongoing orientation and inservice about abuse and neglect:

- §483.13(c), F226—The facility must develop and operationalize policies and procedures for screening and training employees, protection of residents and for the prevention, identification, investigation, and reporting of abuse, neglect, mistreatment, and misappropriation of property. The purpose is to assure that the facility is doing all that is within its control to prevent occurrences.

- Guidelines §483.13(c), F226—The facility must develop and implement policies and procedures that include the seven components: screening, training, prevention, identification, investigation, protection and reporting/response.

Managing cardiac emergencies

The standards of care hold nurses accountable for maintaining competence needed to perform procedures that are part of the job responsibility. CPR is a procedure that is occasionally needed in the care of the residents.

The American Heart Association and American Red Cross offer classes for health professionals to teach cardiopulmonary resuscitation and other emergency procedures. The procedures taught by these agencies constitute the standard of care for emergencies in which the resident is choking on food or a foreign body, or if respirations and/or circulation have ceased.

Brain death begins within four minutes of the time of cardiac or respiratory arrest, or occlusion of the airway. Because of the narrow time frame, nurses must begin emergency resuscitation procedures while awaiting the arrival of an ambulance. Nurses are expected to maintain proficiency in the skills needed to manage the resident pending ambulance arrival, and for complete and accurate documentation of the event. This means accepting the professional responsibility for keeping CPR certification current. Although this is the nurse's professional responsibility, the facility may also be liable under the respondeat superior doctrine if the nurses mismanage an emergency. This is an unnecessary, avoidable risk.

Nursing responsibilities

The information below is based on a state board of nursing position paper on nursing management of emergencies in long-term care facilities:[3]

- Whether CPR is initiated or not, the nurse may be held accountable if the nurse failed to meet standards of care to assure the safety of the resident, prior to a cardiac or respiratory arrest such as:

  - Failure to monitor the resident's physiologic status

  - Failure to document changes in the resident's status and to adjust the plan of care based on the resident assessment

  - Failure to implement appropriate interventions that might be required to stabilize a client's condition, such as reporting changes in the resident's status to the resident's primary care provider and obtaining appropriate orders

  - Failure to implement procedures or protocols that could reasonably be expected to improve the resident's outcome

Documentation

After assessment of the resident is completed and appropriate interventions taken, the nurse must accurately document the circumstances and the assessment of the resident in the medical record. Important documentation elements include:

- Description of the discovery of the resident.

- Any treatment of the resident that was undertaken.

- The findings for each of the assessment elements outlined in the standards.

- All individuals notified of the resident's status (e.g., 911, the healthcare provider, the administrator of the facility, family, coroner, etc.).

- Any directions that were provided to staff or others during the assessment/treatment of the resident.

- The results of any communications.

- Presence or absence of witnesses.

- Documentation should be adequate to give a clear picture of the situation and all of the actions taken or not taken on behalf of the resident.

- Even if a decision not to initiate CPR was appropriate, failure to document can result in an action against a nurse's license by the board of nursing. Furthermore, lack of documentation places the nurse at a disadvantage should the nurse be required to explain the circumstances of the resident's death.

- Nurses should be aware that actions documented at the time of death provide a much more credible defense than needing to prove actions not appropriately documented were actually taken.

Equipment malfunction

Emergency equipment is not used regularly. It tends to disappear. Parts become separated. Supplies such as portable oxygen and suction are not always properly maintained. Because of this, facilities should consider a checklist system for regularly monitoring the emergency box (or crash cart) and supplies. The contents of your emergency box are recommended by the quality assurance committee. List each item on a checklist and designate a time (every shift, every day, every week, etc.) for personnel to check the emergency box against the list. Make sure equipment with moving parts (such as oxygen and suction) are properly assembled and in working order. Check to be sure the portable oxygen source contains sufficient oxygen. Drugs are maintained separately, and are usually kept in a locked medication room. At a minimum, your emergency box should contain:

- Gloves and other personal protective equipment (PPE)

- Pocket mask with oxygen inlet and antireflux valves (extra valves should be stocked elsewhere in the facility; the valve is discarded and replaced after each use)

- Extension tubing for oxygen (connect pocket mask to tank)

- Portable suction machine

- Variety of suction catheters

- Oral airways

- Backboard/CPR board

- Tape

- Assortment of dressings and bandages

- Automatic defibrillator, with pads and supplies, if available

- Portable oxygen source

- Assortment of oxygen masks (face and tracheostomy) and oxygen tubing

- Oxygen precautions sign(s)

Use of oxygen in an emergency

Oxygen is necessary for life. Some diseases and conditions prevent enough oxygen from nourishing the body's tissues, so supplemental oxygen is administered. Oxygen is a basic need at the lowest level of Maslow's hierarchy of needs. Needs at the lower levels must be fulfilled before needs at the higher levels become important. Since the need for oxygen is a low-level need, the resident who is having trouble breathing cannot focus on much else. Oxygen is a prescription item, and a physician's order is necessary to administer it to a resident. Your facility policies may permit nurses to administer oxygen in an emergency, but if a general standing order is eventually implemented for a resident, physician notification and a proper order are necessary.

Simple formula for determining duration of oxygen cylinder use

Number of minutes the cylinder will last = Gauge pressure in pounds per square inch (psi) minus 200 (which is the safe residual pressure) times the cylinder constant (see below) divided by the liter flow per minute.

Cylinder Constants
D = 0.16
E = 0.28
G = 2.41
H = 3.14
K = 3.14
M = 1.56

Example:
Determine the life of an E cylinder that has a pressure of 2000 psi on the pressure gauge. The flow rate is 10 liters per minute.

$$\frac{(2000-200) \times 0.28}{10} = \frac{504}{10} = 50.4 \text{ minutes}$$

If the number of minutes exceeds 60, you can convert to hours by dividing by 60. For example, you determine that a cylinder will last 135 minutes. $135 \div 60 = 2$ hours and 15 minutes.

Oxygen delivery devices

Many different types of oxygen administration devices are used. The nasal cannula is most commonly used in long-term care facilities to provide oxygen at low-liter flows. In a cardiac emergency, high-liter flows are necessary. Because of this, oxygen masks are used in emergencies. A mask should never be used with liter flows below five because it may cause rebreathing of the resident's exhaled carbon dioxide, and has a smothering effect, which is very frightening to the resident who is struggling to breathe.

The nonrebreathing mask is a modification of the simple oxygen mask. The nonrebreathing mask is used for residents with severe hypoxemia. The mask has one way plastic flaps on the sides. Exhaled air escapes through the flaps, but outside air cannot enter. A reservoir bag is connected to the bottom of the mask. The combination of bag and mask increase the amount of oxygen delivered to the resident. If the system is working properly, the bag will be inflated at all times. It should not collapse more than halfway during inhalation.

Oxygen delivery systems

In some facilities, oxygen is piped in through an internal system in the walls. The flow meter is connected to a wall adapter. Oxygen is delivered when the flow meter is turned on. Some units have more than one adapter. Oxygen is always color coded with a green label in the United States. Read carefully when initiating oxygen through a piped-in system. Make sure you are using the correct adapter and plug. In facilities with piped in oxygen systems, small portable oxygen cylinders are used for transporting residents from one area to another, and may be used in emergencies in hallways or other areas without a piped-in source.

Most long-term care facilities use oxygen cylinders or concentrators. The oxygen concentrator converts room air to oxygen and delivers it to the resident. Oxygen also comes in a liquid canister. The canister delivers a higher concentration of oxygen than a concentrator, but is portable and convenient. It does not require electricity to operate. It is quiet compared with a concentrator, which has an electric motor and makes a humming noise. Liquid and cylinder oxygen is more expensive than using a concentrator. Generally speaking, a concentrator will not convert room air to oxygen in liter flows over five. Therefore, use a portable tank or liquid canister in an emergency. Do not use a concentrator.

Flow meters

The flow of oxygen to the resident is regulated by a flow meter that shows how many liters of oxygen are being delivered each minute. Increase the flow by turning the knob clockwise, and decrease the flow by turning it counterclockwise. Flow meters come in various sizes and shapes, but all work the same way. However, the various size cylinders use different gauges.

If you are setting up a cylinder, make sure the gauges fit. Read the label on the flow meter to ensure it is for use on oxygen tanks. In this case, you cannot depend on color coding. Colors are not always consistent with flow meters, as they are for oxygen cylinders and other parts.

Oxygen regulator fires

In 2006, the Food and Drug Administration (FDA) issued a warning about safety hazards associated with the washers and gaskets used in oxygen regulators. FDA has received reports in which regulators used with oxygen cylinders have burned or exploded, in some cases injuring personnel. Some of the incidents occurred during emergency medical use or during routine equipment checks. FDA and The National Institute for Occupational Safety and Health (NIOSH) believe that improper use of gaskets/washers in these regulators was a major factor in both the ignition and severity of the fires, although there are likely other contributing factors.

Two types of washers, referred to as CGA 870 seals, are commonly used to create the seal at the juncture of the cylinder valve and regulator interface: The type recommended by many regulator manufacturers is a metal-bound elastomeric sealing washer that is designed for multiple use applications. The other common type, often supplied free-of-charge with refilled oxygen cylinders, is a plastic (usually Nylon®) crush gasket suitable for single use applications. When used more than once, the nylon crush gaskets require increased pressure to tighten the unit at each use. (The unit is assembled and tightened by hand.) As the wear on the gasket increases, a wrench is necessary to obtain a proper seal. Unfortunately, the pressure from the wrench increases the risk of damage to both the gasket and the regulator. Leakage of oxygen across the surface of the gasket increases the risk of spontaneous ignition. To prevent injury, FDA and NIOSH recommend:

- Using crush gaskets one time only, then replacing them.

- Cracking cylinder valves to allow the escape of oxygen before attaching a regulator to the cylinder.

- Using the sealing gasket recommended by the manufacturer.

- Inspecting the regulator and CGA 870 seal before attaching it to the valve to ensure the correct gasket is used and it is in good condition.

- Make sure the gasket, valve, and regulator are free from grease and oil.

- Tighten the T-handle firmly by hand; avoid wrenches and tools.

- Open the post valve slowly. If gas escapes at the juncture of the regulator and valve, quickly close the valve. Verify the regulator is properly attached and the gasket is properly placed and in good condition.

For additional information and FDA medical device notifications, go to *www.fda.gov/cdrh/ safety.html.*

Pressure gauge

The pressure gauge shows how much oxygen is in the cylinder. It is connected to the flow meter on an oxygen cylinder. Oxygen is measured in pounds. Check the gauge regularly and make sure another unit is available before the cylinder is empty. Most facilities consider cylinders empty when the pressure reaches 500 pounds. You may have to estimate how long a cylinder will last based on the cylinder size and the number of liters per minute of oxygen use.

Humidifiers

Some facilities attach humidifiers to the oxygen equipment. Humidification is not necessary in liter flows below five. Do not delay emergency oxygen to look for a humidifier. Over a prolonged period of time, dry oxygen may become uncomfortable at high-liter flows, but this is not an issue in the early stages of an emergency when seconds count. Use of oxygen humidifiers is a controversial subject, and some facilities have eliminated them entirely.

The humidifier moistens the oxygen for comfort and prevents drying of the mucous membranes in the nose, mouth, and lungs. The humidifier bottle screws into a male adapter on the flow meter. Oxygen passes through the water in the humidifier to collect moisture before it reaches the resident. The cannula or mask plugs into a male adapter on the side of the humidifier. Never use tap water to fill a humidifier. Inhalation of tap water is associated with an increased incidence of Legionnaire's disease. Sterile distilled water should always be used. Keep the water level in the humidifier at or above the "minimum fill" line on the bottle.

When the system is functioning correctly, water in the humidifier will bubble. Oxygen will not exit the tubing into the mask or cannula if the tubing is kinked or obstructed. If this occurs, pressure builds up in the unit and discharges through a pressure relief valve. When setting up a humidifier, check the valve to make sure it works by turning the oxygen on and pinching the connecting tubing.

Preparing the oxygen cylinder

Supplies needed:

- Oxygen cylinder.

- Wrench, depending on type of flow meter used.

- Handle or wrench for opening the cylinder valve.

- Flow meter to fit the cylinder.

- Sterile humidifier bottle, if used.

- Sterile distilled water for humidifier (or use sterile prefilled humidifier).

- Tubing and delivery device.

- Obtain the cylinder. Check the color and read the label to verify the contents.

- Transport the cylinder chained to a wheeled dolly.

- Position the cylinder upright on the dolly, upright in a base, or chained to the wall.

- Stand to the side. Remove the metal or plastic cap, or wrapper protecting the outlet.

- Attach the handle to the cylinder. Crack the main valve for one second. Close the valve.

- Position the cylinder valve gasket on the regulator port.

- Check the regulator. Turn the knob to make sure the regulator port is closed.

- Align the two holes in the outlet with the two pins in the regulator, or thread the nut onto the male adapter on the outlet. Tighten the T-screw for the pin yolk, or use a wrench to tighten the threaded outlet. If you are using a small cylinder-type regulator, a Teflon "O" ring must be in place or the connection will leak.

- Turn the cylinder on and check the pressure gauge. The cylinder should be full. Listen for air leaks. If you hear a leak, turn the cylinder off, remove the regulator, then reapply.

- Attach the humidifier filled with sterile distilled water, tubing, and delivery device, if used.

- Post the oxygen precautions sign(s) according to facility policy.

Discontinuing an oxygen cylinder

Your facility will have policies and procedures for cleaning and storing oxygen cylinders after they are used. A portable emergency cylinder or transport cylinder may be used for a brief time, then returned to the storage area for reuse. Before storing an oxygen cylinder, you must turn the oxygen off. When this is done, a certain amount of oxygen remains in the gauges. Bleeding the cylinder is a simple, yet essential procedure that ensures no oxygen remains in the gauges. Bleed the gauge by turning the oxygen supply from the cylinder to the flow meter off (by turning the valve on top). Next, turn the flow meter on. Although the cylinder is turned off, the flow meter will rise momentarily, then the liter flow will drop to zero. This removes the remaining free oxygen from the gauges so the tank is safe to store.

General standards of care for administering oxygen in an emergency

Do not delay mouth to pocket mask resuscitation while waiting for portable oxygen to arrive. Initiate mouth to mask ventilation immediately. Connect the oxygen to the inlet on the side of the face mask when it arrives, using an extension tubing. Run the oxygen at high liter flows, usually 12 to 15 liters per minute, or according to facility policy.

To meet the standard of care for administering oxygen safely:

- Follow facility policies for administering oxygen by standing order; notify the physician of the change in the resident's condition as soon as possible. Prepare to transfer the resident to the emergency department according to facility policy.

- Notify the physician immediately of deterioration in condition, or follow facility policy for transporting the resident to the emergency department via 911 ambulance.

- Before initiating oxygen therapy, check the resident's room to make sure it is safe for oxygen delivery.

- Oxygen is always color coded with a green label or green tank in the United States. Never use a tank or wall inlet with a different color. Read carefully.

- The parts for an oxygen system fit together readily. If they do not fit, double check the system to ensure you are using oxygen and that the parts are for oxygen therapy. Make sure you are using the correct adapter and plug. Never attempt to modify an oxygen apparatus to fit a tank or wall outlet. If the connectors do not fit, the device is not intended for use. Never bypass or modify parts to make them fit together.

- Never force the flow meter into the wall or cylinder when assembling an oxygen unit. Forcing the flow meter may cause a valve to stick in an open position, causing oxygen to leak out.

- Obtain an oxygen cylinder or canister for emergencies. Never use a concentrator.

  - Never use an oxygen mask with a concentrator.

  - Never use an oxygen cannula in an emergency. Use a mask with high-liter flows.

  - Never use grease or oil on oxygen cylinder connections.

  - Transport oxygen cylinders carefully. They should be chained to a carrier during transport. Avoid dropping them.

- Secure oxygen cylinders or canisters in a base or chain them to a carrier or the wall. Avoid dropping the tank. By itself, oxygen is not highly explosive. However, cylinders can explode if the unit is dropped and the valve is damaged.

- Post "Oxygen in Use" signs over the bed and on the door of the room, or according to facility policy. The sign should list warnings, such as not smoking.

- Remove all sources of ignition from the room, including matches and lighters, cigarettes, and some electrical appliances.

- Assess the resident's vital signs every 15 minutes, or according to need.

- Assess and document capillary refill and pulse oximeter readings upon initiation of oxygen therapy. Continue to check these periodically while oxygen is being used.

- If using piped-in oxygen, gently pull the flow meter to ensure it will not fall out. If the humidifier is not used, screw the triangular adapter ("Christmas tree") to the bottom of the flow meter. Connect the tubing to the point of the triangle.

- Turn the oxygen on; set at the designated flow rate by adjusting the knob on the flow meter.

- Check the flow of oxygen by placing your hand in front of inlet and feeling for the flow of oxygen.

- Position the mask over the resident's nose, mouth, and chin. Mold the metal band at the top of the mask to the resident's nose.

- Slip the elastic strap behind the resident's head. Tighten the adjustment so the strap is secure, but not too tight.

- Elevate the head of the bed when the resident is receiving oxygen.

- Dress the resident in a cotton gown and cover him or her with a cotton blanket. Avoid using wool and synthetic blankets and clothing. The resident's gown and linen on the bed absorb extra oxygen from the air. Extra oxygen may cause objects to burn much faster than they normally would.

- Some facilities remove the call signal and replace it with a bell that is used manually. The call signal may cause a spark.

- If oxygen equipment makes an unusual noise, take corrective action or notify the appropriate person immediately. If you suspect a cylinder or wall outlet is leaking, remove the resident from the room and close the door.

Other considerations for oxygen use

Learn how to turn off oxygen in case of a fire emergency. Piped-in oxygen may be turned off at a zone valve in the hallway. Cylinders, canisters, and concentrators must be turned off at the unit. Facility personnel must learn and follow facility policies and procedures for transporting and evacuating residents needing continuous oxygen in an emergency. Follow infection control precautions when caring for residents using oxygen, such as keeping the tubing, mask, or cannula covered when not in use. Keep the tubing and delivery system off the floor. Follow all other facility policies and procedures for oxygen safety.

Managing noncardiac emergencies

The facility must have detailed written plans, policies, and procedures for managing all potential emergencies and disasters. In some states, an emergency manual is required, listing state-specified emergency procedures and inservice requirements. The facility must make provisions for teaching employees their role and responsibility in various emergencies. Review and update all policies and procedures at least annually. Consider using "mock codes" and similar hands-on training, by implementing unannounced staff drills to familiarize personnel with emergency procedures.

The physician should be notified immediately if the resident's condition shows signs of significant deterioration, respiratory distress, or abnormal vital signs. If one nurse is on duty, notify the physician as soon as you can safely do so. Follow his or her orders for treatment. Notify the nearest relative or responsible party when you can safely do so. Many facilities have policies permitting nurses to call 911 for immediate hospital transport, bypassing the need for physician orders. If this is the case, concentrate on getting the resident to the hospital, then notify the physician and responsible party. Use a 911 ambulance in a life or death emergency, not a transfer service. If the resident is not transferred to the hospital, continue monitoring for at least 24 hours or until the emergency is completely resolved and the resident is stable.

Document the entire situation carefully and completely, including exact times for changes in condition, observations, notifications, vital signs, and emergency diagnostic tests and care provided. Document the resident's response. Complete a separate incident report, if appropriate, and according to facility policy. If an incident is of a serious nature, it should be investigated by or under the direction of the director of nurses or quality assurance committee. Some incidents also must be reported to state authorities. Follow facility policies and state law.

Incident reports

An incident is an unusual occurrence or event that interrupts normal procedures or causes a crisis. It may or may not result in an injury to a resident or worker. An incident report is a form that is completed for each accident or unusual event or occurrence in a long-term care facility. The incident report describes what happened and contains other important information. Each facility has policies, procedures, and forms for incident reporting. Some facilities use a separate form for medication-related incidents. Each state also has requirements for reporting incidents to the regulatory body. Reportable incidents usually include those in which a resident is seriously injured or dies. The definition of what constitutes "serious" also varies. In some states, fractures are considered serious, whereas in others they are not. Know and follow your facility policies and state laws for incident reports.

The ultimate goal of incident and adverse event reports is to use them for root cause analysis. This process is used to answer questions such as:

- What happened?

- Why did it happen?

- What can be done so it does not happen again?

Nursing responsibilities

Nurses are accountable for:

- Being familiar with facility policies and procedures for incidents, accidents, and emergencies

- Being familiar with and implementing the applicable standards of care for emergencies

- Maintaining competence in emergency procedures

- Being familiar with each resident's code or advance directive status, knowing where to find this information quickly in an emergency, and knowing how to interpret and when to apply the information

- Monitoring the resident's physiologic status

- Documenting changes in the resident's status

- Adjusting the plan of care based on changes in resident status and assessment

- Implementing appropriate interventions to stabilize a resident's condition

- Reporting changes in the resident's status to the primary care provider, obtaining, and following appropriate orders

- Reporting changes in the resident's status to the responsible party

- Implementing procedures or protocols that could reasonably be expected to improve the resident's outcome

- Following facility policies and procedures for immediate 911 transport in the event of a life-threatening emergency

Take incident reporting seriously. Completing an incident report and documenting on the medical record may seem redundant. However, do not cut corners. Be thorough and concise. The incident report for an accident or injury such as a fall should include:

- Circumstances of the incident

- Date, time, location, shift, unit

- Witnesses, staff and resident accounts of the incident

- Interventions taken to care for the resident immediately after the incident

- Notifications made as a result of an incident

- Resident symptoms prior to the incident

- Vital signs and observations made after the incident

- Resident activity at the time of the incident

- Injuries/medical problems associated with the incident

- Environmental hazards or faulty equipment contributing to the incident

- Presence of any new incident risk factors

- Corrective actions taken to reduce the likelihood of another incident

Nursing actions to take if an incident occurs:

- Immediately after the incident, the nurse should:

  - Get help (if needed)

  - Provide emergency care to stabilize the resident; take the appropriate action

- Notify the appropriate individuals:

- Facility administrative personnel, such as director of nursing and administrator (follow facility policy for notification)

- Physician

- Resident's family or responsible party

- State agency, if incident falls within mandatory reporting guidelines

If the incident involves a piece of medical equipment, know your reporting responsibilities under the Safe Medical Devices Act of 1990. Each healthcare facility is required to have a designated individual to report to FDA, using a special form.

- Complete an incident report:

  - The incident report is used to alert administrative personnel to problems, to gather data, and to provide quality assurance information for studies and statistics designed to reduce incidents and injuries. Avoid referring to the incident report elsewhere in your documentation. Referring to it makes it part of the medical record.

- Make sure all information on the incident report is legible:

  - Avoid referring to incident reports to visitors, family members, and nonemployees.

  - Avoid documenting your opinions or assumptions on the incident report. Document only facts.

  - Avoid mentioning action to prevent recurrence in the incident report, such as having a piece of equipment repaired. However, if a single piece of potentially faulty equipment is mentioned in the incident report, it is appropriate to note immediate action taken. For example, you suspect a bed rail is not holding securely. Note that the resident was placed in another bed until the bed rails can be inspected by maintenance.

  - Never refer to an investigation or report to an insurance company on the incident report or medical record.

  - Avoid making statements that place blame. This is a personal judgment. State the facts objectively.

  - Complete the entire incident report during the shift on which the incident occurred.

  - Use black ink.

  - Document the particulars of the incident, including date, time, and notifications.

Make sure the times are accurate.

- Avoid leaving blanks in data that may be questioned later. Be objective and avoid speculation. Describe what you saw or were told by the resident and witnesses.

- State the names of witnesses. Some facilities do not want addresses and phone numbers recorded, feeling that this provides helpful information to plaintiff attorneys. Follow your facility policy.

- Never ask a family member or visitor to complete or sign an incident report. Doing this entitles them to a copy of the report. If they insist on completing an incident report, do not provide a facility form. Have them write a statement on a piece of paper and sign it. Forward it to the appropriate administrative person.

- Never alter or falsify a medical record. Complete your documentation on incidents and injuries during the shift in which they occurred. Avoid late entry charting, if possible.

• Initiate ongoing monitoring and plan for aftercare:

- Update the care plan.

- Pass the information on in your shift report.

- Provide follow-up monitoring and care.

- Initiate the proper forms for monitoring vital signs, neurological checks, etc.

- Document postinjury assessment, intervention, and monitoring.

- Document notifications.

- Include your signature and title.

- Monitor the resident every shift, or more often if necessary, until the incident is resolved and the resident has been stable for more than 24 hours. Follow facility policy for vital signs and neurological checks. When the incident is resolved, make a notation in the nurses' notes describing the resident's condition related to injuries incurred in the incident.

• Initiate an investigation. (This investigation is initiated/completed by nurses on the unit, according to facility policy. Investigating incidents is a learning experience for staff and charge nurses and the results are very useful to resident care and services.)

- Identify the incident or adverse event

- Determine priorities for investigation and time frame; emergencies or environmental problems may require immediate investigation

- Determine who will investigate the incident

- Gather information

- Determine the chronology of the incident; investigate the time line and potential precipitating and contributory factors

- Determine whether a pattern exists

- Analyze the data; turn raw data into information, information into knowledge, and knowledge into an action plan

- Document your findings and maintain a record of the investigation and outcome

- Implement the plan

- Keep a quality assurance log or other record to look for trends in accidents that can be anticipated and avoided.

Documentation

In most facilities you will chronicle the incident in the nurses' notes without mentioning the incident report. Some facilities do not want facts of an incident stated on the medical record. The theory is that the medical record is for resident injury and care issues. The incident report focuses on other details and circumstances. Assuming your facility requires documentation of the incident in the nursing notes, do so after assessment of the resident is completed, appropriate interventions taken, and the resident stabilized. Important elements of this documentation are:

- Description of discovery of the resident

- Treatment provided

- Assessment findings

- Notifications (e.g., 911, the healthcare provider, the administrator or director of nursing, family, coroner, etc.)

- Results of communications

- Explanation of directions provided to staff or others during the assessment/treatment of the resident

- Presence or absence of witnesses; witness statements

- Documentation should provide an articulate picture of the situation and actions taken on behalf of the resident

Potential personal legal exposure

Even if nursing decisions and actions are appropriate, failure to document can result in untoward actions by the state health department, by the board of nursing, or in a civil lawsuit. Absence of documentation places the nurse and facility at a disadvantage if they are required to describe the circumstances of a serious injury or death. Documentation from the time of the event is often viewed as much more credible than late entry charting (which may be viewed as self-serving), verbal statements, or testimony at a trial or hearing.

If you are involved in an incident in which you believe you have personal liability, you may wish to notify your malpractice insurer of the event. Remember that accurate and concise incident reporting offers a measure of protection as well as a means for analyzing trends to reduce incidents and injuries in the future. Providing the data on incidents provides an opportunity for teamwork and commitment. As you can see, the report has many useful purposes and completing it is much more than an exercise in paper compliance!

Follow up on adverse events or incidents

A successful nurse manager must know what is happening on the resident care units from day to day. Being aware of incidents and adverse events and taking the appropriate action is critical to reducing legal exposure. The primary purpose of the incident report is to communicate this information in one succinct document that can be reviewed by many individuals.

The details of an incident are recorded in the resident's medical record. Medication errors may require a special type of incident report. Although falls are the most common adverse events, an incident report should be completed for any abnormal occurrence. Studying the incident reports each day will help you:

- Discover the cause of the fall or other event

- Identify circumstances surrounding the fall, as well as potential contributing causes

- Identify methods of preventing another incident from occurring

- Employing measures to protect staff and the facility against legal action

Incident investigation

All incidents should be reviewed, investigated, and analyzed in a timely manner. Astute managers will use the data on incident reports to track, trend, and profile incidents on the unit. At a minimum, review and look at incident reports cumulatively to see whether you can identify preventable patterns in the:

- Time of day

  - Analyzing trends for the time when most incidents occur causes the manager to look at staffing and other factors (such as whether more incidents occur at meal-time, when staff are occupied or off the unit), leading to changes in numbers of staff and other routines.

- Day of week

  - Some days are perpetually short-staffed. Knowing that shortage of staff increases incidents on certain days may effect positive changes in staffing.

- Nature of incident

  - Managers look for patterns in the nature and type of incident. For example, if there are patterns of incidents involving transfers or wet floors, the astute manager will institute changes in procedure to reduce injury.

- Type of incident

  - Does the incident involve an employee, resident, or both? The manager will investigate methods to reduce incidents in this population. If a certain employee is repeatedly involved in incidents, he or she should receive remediation or additional education to prevent future events.

- Environmental factors

  - Reviewing environmental factors may surprise you. Although most incidents occur indoors, in a temperature controlled environment, you may find confounding factors. For example, on a carpeted floor surface, nonslip soles may cause residents to stumble. A shiny floor may reflect light, causing a glare and making it difficult for residents to see. Alternating light and dark tiles may alter the residents' perception. One facility discovered that some residents perceived dark tiles to be holes. The residents tried to step over the holes, resulting in loss of balance and falls.

- Notifications

  - Typically the incident report will list notifications made as a result of the incident. The manager will audit this area to ensure that the physician, responsible party, or other notifications are made consistently. Failure to communicate is enormously problematic.

- Follow-up

  - The perceptive manager will use the incident reports as a means of following up on staff investigation and postincident monitoring. Monitoring continues until resolution of the incident. For example, an unwitnessed fall or known head injury is followed on all shifts for at least 72 hours to rule out subdural hematoma.

Quality assurance is given various titles within the healthcare facility. Regardless of the title, the quality assurance committee should take an active interest in incident reduction. If a unit or facility has a pattern of incidents, the committee will review potential contributing factors and act on them through education or other methods of risk reduction. Most nursing personnel view completion of incident reports as "paper compliance." All papers generated by facility staff are tools for communication, and incident reports are no exception. The quality assurance committee will take them very seriously.

Witness statements

Getting eyewitness and staff information is an important part of your investigation. However, in some situations employees make incorrect assumptions, such as believing that talking loudly to a hearing-impaired resident constitutes verbal abuse. Grammatical errors, misspellings, and incomplete sentence structure usually do not project a positive or professional image of facility personnel. In a court of law the defense attorney must try to defend the employee statements. Statements regarding "short staffing" can be particularly damaging. If documentation of these interviews or written witness statements are subjective or point blame at someone or something, you may find the investigation information used against you. Verbal and written statements may contain indefensible or irrelevant information.

Because of the potential problems with taking written employee statements, you may wish to consider verbal employee interviews. Although interviewing is more time-consuming, it enables you to obtain accurate information. Write a summary of the relevant information, then ask the employee to review it and sign it to verify its accuracy. Once an employee statement has been written, avoid asking the individual to rewrite it. Rewriting suggests the investigator was attempting to get the employee to change his or her story, or was trying to influence the documented information. If it is necessary to add information, do so by using an addendum page. Written statements must never be destroyed. Destruction of records and statements suggests a cover-up or wrongdoing.

Check with your risk-management department or legal counsel regarding a format to use to document the investigation. Written information and documentation are usually considered permanent. The rules of discovery in your state may permit opposing counsel to obtain all documentation and incident investigation information. Typically, employee statements are not protected.

Risk-reduction programs

Facilities should consider investigating all incidents, even if there are no injuries. Develop or test recognized resident risk-assessment tools that meet the needs of your facility population when developing effective systemwide side rail and restraint reduction programs. No single assessment tool is appropriate for all facilities. Several different assessment tools may be needed to meet the needs of your resident population. However, you should limit the number of assessments for a singular purpose (such as fall risk or restraint reduction) as much as possible to avoid confusing staff.

All healthcare facilities have a risk-management process. Incident reports with injuries involving potential liability or those with high risk of legal exposure must be referred to the risk-management department immediately. Expect the risk manager to interview witnesses and gather additional information.

This is done to protect all parties involved. It should not be perceived as a punitive process done for the purpose of "getting" the involved employee. In fact, studies have revealed that many incidents are caused by systematic errors instead of employee negligence. However, reporting all incidents and accidents is essential despite the potential for personal consequences. The root cause analysis will reveal whether an organization or systemic failure or breakdown caused or contributed to the incident.

Need for individualized care

One reason that formal incident and fall-prevention programs are unsuccessful is that they take a "one "size fits all" approach. Individualize incident and fall prevention measures to the residents' problems and needs. It goes without saying that no two residents are exactly alike. Certain approaches are generic to all residents, and should not be considered part of the individualized plan. When every fall-prevention care plan says, "call light in reach," and "remind resident to call for help," your plan is not individualized.

A review of the MDSs may reveal that the residents at greatest risk have short- and long-term memory loss. An individualized approach that says, "Remind the resident to use the call signal" is likely to be forgotten by the resident, and the MDS verifies this fact. When a resident falls, nurse managers say, "But we had a fall prevention plan in place." Did you, really? Was it generic or individualized? A generic plan may be the problem.

Evaluate your plans before serious injury occurs. For success, the fall and incident prevention plan must be personalized to each resident's individual problems and needs. This seems obvious, but in the real world it does not always happen. Review the residents' incident prevention plans. See whether they are generic (such as listing the approaches above) or individualized. Then check to see whether the planned approaches have been implemented. Look for proof of that implementation. This is exactly the type of audit that a medical-legal reviewer will do if your chart is involved in litigation. You will be either surprised or pleased at the results. (Surprise occurs if you find generic, "one size fits all" plans. You will be pleased if you find individualized plans. You will be surprised if you find no documentation that fall prevention has been implemented, and pleased if you do.) In any event, this review is an excellent way to evaluate and improve the effectiveness of your fall prevention program, and gives you one perspective on the medical-legal review.

The next step in evaluating your program is to look at the risk-assessment tool you are using. Make sure the assessment means more than paper compliance. Then:

- Ask the nurses for their interpretation of the residents' risk status, and how their care changes when a resident's risk increases.

- Compare the questions on the tool with the needs of the residents. Do the questions identify specific medical problems that increase fall risk? Residents have a variety of problems and needs.

- Make sure the tool you use is appropriate for your facility population. If a tool identifies a resident as being at high risk, make sure the interventions implemented (and listed on the care plan) are aggressive and match the degree of risk.

- Avoid using routine, low-risk interventions for a high-risk resident. The monitoring and protection to the resident should increase proportionately with the degree of risk.

- Implement interventions as soon as the risk factor is known. Do not wait until an incident or untoward event occurs!

To err is human

In 1999, the Institute of Medicine (IOM) Committee on Quality of Care in America released a report called, *To Err Is Human*.[4] The report identifies major areas of patient injury and death. Common errors are:[5]

- Diagnostic

  - Error or delay in diagnosis

- Failure to employ indicated tests

- Use of outmoded tests or therapy

- Failure to act on results of monitoring or testing

- Treatment

    - Error in the performance of an operation, procedure, or test

    - Error in administering the treatment

    - Error in the dose or method of using a drug

    - Avoidable delay in treatment or in responding to an abnormal test

    - Inappropriate (not indicated) care

- Preventive

    - Failure to provide prophylactic treatment

    - Inadequate monitoring or follow-up of treatment

- Other

    - Failure of communication

    - Equipment failure

    - Other system failure

One of the report's main conclusions (and one that must be learned in long-term care) is that most errors are not the result of individual recklessness. Most often, errors result from faulty systems, processes, and conditions that cause employees to make mistakes or fail to prevent them. The report contends that it is best to prevent mistakes by designing the health system to make it safer; and to make it easier to do a job right and more difficult to do something wrong. They note that when an error occurs, blaming an individual does little to make the system safer and prevent someone else from committing the same error.

A commentary about the IOM report in the *Harvard Healthcare Review* describes how one physician risk manager contacted NASA to learn how to improve quality in his hospital.[6] The following is excerpted from this story, but take the time to read and motivate yourself by this powerful safety message:

"In response to the question, "How do you get good enough to get to the moon?" Guy Cohen had no one-liners to offer me. He didn't say, 'Report Cards,' or 'Market Forces,' or 'Incentive Pay,' or even

'Accountability.' In fact, as I recall it, not one of those words came up in the time we spent together. His views of human nature, organizations, systems, and change would not permit one-line answers."

The writer makes an analogy between a serious rocket problem that was almost overlooked and a medication error with the potential for patient injury or death. When asked how the hospital would handle a similar incident, he explains that they would discipline or fire a nurse.

The NASA administrator's response was, "Then you will never be safe." The risk manager concludes, "I think the point is clear. You have to be very smart to design a rocket right, and even smarter to figure out what happened and correct it when something goes wrong. However, you have to be even smarter still to design and lead the supra-ordinate system—not the system of work, but the system of leadership and management in which the work system will thrive or wither."[7]

The IOM report emphasizes that the healthcare system must learn from mistakes. Think of how this applies to residents with a history of falls. Most residents who fall have a history of recurrent falls before a fracture or other serious injury occurs. Your actions immediately after a resident falls have the potential to mitigate the fall risk. Immediately after a fall, you will assess, stabilize, and treat the resident, make notifications, document the incident, and complete reports. Next, you will establish a monitoring system for vital signs, neurological checks, and other data as appropriate.

This is where nursing action commonly ends. Do not stop here! The actions you take from here on out will probably affect the likelihood that the resident will fall again.
Based on the present fall, the resident's fall risk has just increased. Completing your documentation and returning to your other responsibilities will not affect this resident's risk of future falls. You may need to request assistance in caring for other residents so you can complete the fall-related care. Doing so will reduce the risk of personal liability, as well as reducing the facility's legal exposure. Now you must investigate the incident and take steps to reduce future fall risk. This cannot wait until the next care conference. It must be done now.

Most falls occur as the result of multiple factors. Some are environmental, but others are intrinsic (medical, personal). Identify and mitigate as many risk factors as possible. Consider conditions such as osteoporosis or history of previous fracture, use of anticoagulant drugs, or problems that will worsen a potential fall. Social factors are probably not significant, but may be worth considering. For example, knowing the type and size of the bed the resident formerly slept in, and patterns of social behavior (such as noncompliance or need for independence) may give you insight into fall risks and behaviors. Consider the activity the resident was engaged in at the time of the fall. Reevaluate the risk factors. Complete another fall risk-assessment tool after each fall. If the resident was found on the floor after an unknown period of time, determine why he or she was not found sooner. Determine whether unmet needs contributed to the fall. This is commonly true in residents who cannot communicate their needs.

Evaluate the orthostatic blood pressure.[8] This is an important, and often omitted, step. Evaluate the medication regimen. Research has shown that fall risk increases when residents take four or more medications.[9] Assess the resident for signs and symptoms of acute illness, which accounts for almost 25% of falls.[10] Many falls occur during the first few days of admission, when the resident is new and unfamiliar with the environment. Likewise, staff are not familiar with the resident's problems and needs. Identify as many risks as possible. Ask for ideas from nursing assistants on strategies for reducing risk. Determine what care plan changes need to be implemented. Notify the resident and responsible party of the results of the risk assessment. Collaborate on prevention strategies. Be candid when discussing quality of life versus risks of preventive care, such as restraints, alternatives, and assistive mobility devices.

Note that all falls cannot be prevented, but the facility will do all they can to reduce the risk of fall-related injuries. Determine whether fear of falling will affect the resident's future behavior, activities, mobility, or family attitudes. If so, address the fears in the plan of care. Develop and implement a plan that modifies as many risk factors as possible, based on your analysis of the incident. Implement multiple risk-reduction strategies, and modify the environment to further reduce the risk. Communicate with other staff and keep them apprised of approaches to use in care of the resident.

Individualize the plan to your assessment data. Generic approaches that are used regularly in the care of all residents are probably not appropriate, and need not be listed. List approaches that are assessment-based and likely to be effective. Whenever possible, initiate a system of documentation that reflects use of the nursing process[11] and is individualized to the resident's needs. Develop, maintain, and evaluate a format for documentation that facilitates desired outcomes. Documentation should reflect proactive care. Surprisingly, fall documentation is often reactive. Proactive care recognizes that the resident is at risk for certain complications, so preventive care is provided. Documentation may be done by means of a flow sheet or checklist. It need not be lengthy or narrative. Succinct, focused statements showing individualized care are very effective. Reactive approaches to falls defy nursing ethics and the principles upon which nursing practice is based.[12]

Regularly evaluate the effectiveness of the fall prevention plan, and document the results. Although some falls cannot be prevented, immediate postfall assessment, regular evaluation and individualized risk reduction strategies will most likely reduce the total number of falls and risk of serious injuries.

Learning from errors

Study and learn from incidents and injuries. Instead of automatically blaming individuals, evaluate the system to determine whether it promoted the problem. Determine whether a voluntary reporting system will enhance facility data collection and risk reduction. This type of system focuses on errors that do no or minimal harm. This type of quality assurance program will help identify and correct system weaknesses before serious injury occurs. The IOM also recommends implementing safety systems and promoting a "culture of safety" that focuses on improving reliability and safe care.

Safety should be an explicit organizational goal that is demonstrated by strong leadership. This means incorporating a variety of well-understood safety principles, such as designing jobs and working conditions for safety; standardizing and simplifying equipment, supplies, and processes; and enabling care providers to avoid reliance on memory. Systems for continuously monitoring resident safety must also be created and supported.

Public image when an accident occurs

Facilities are sometimes inclined to cover things up, or to squarely point fingers of blame if an accident or injury occurs. Because of this, the incident is not adequately investigated through root cause analysis, and the accident is repeated! If a serious accident occurs:

- Notify the risk manager/legal counsel.

- Formulate a public relations plan for dealing with potentially adverse publicity in advance; follow the plan.

- Begin an investigation immediately; your initial priority is to interview all involved staff and witnesses.

- Avoid pointing fingers or placing blame.

- In the initial stages of the investigation, avoid making assumptions before all facts are in and analyzed.

- Avoid making promises or accepting blame.

- Apologize, if appropriate. Several states have passed laws stating that apologies cannot be used as the basis for a subsequent lawsuit.[13] Anecdotal evidence has revealed that an apology can persuade a patient or resident not to sue.[14]

- Avoid the appearance of impropriety by withholding information from the resident and family. One person should act as spokesperson. Likewise, information should be given to one family member who can advise the others. Avoid communicating through and with multiple individuals, who each may tell a slightly different story.

- If mechanical or electrical equipment is involved, remove it from service and promptly have it checked by an independent, knowledgeable person. The maintenance workers and manufacturers' representatives are not independent sources.

- If a resident or staff member is seriously injured, make arrangements with social services, pastoral care, mental health, or others to debrief workers and assist them in managing their feelings of pain and loss. Be careful in discussions with counselors and avoid giving out confidential information. Medical and clinical information about the event is probably appropriate only for the quality assurance committee. The counselors may be required to testify in a lawsuit later.

References

1. §483.75(h). State Operations Manual.

2. Zagury CS. Making a difference: Strategic planning for the director of nursing in long term care. The Director. Online. www.nadona.org/media_archive/media/media-238.pdf. Accessed 08/25/04.

3. Texas Board of Nurse Examiners. (2003). Position statements. 15.20 nurses in the management of an unwitnessed arrest in a resident in a long-term care facility. Online. www.bne.state.tx.us/position.htm#15.20

4. Institute of Medicine. (1999). To Err Is Human. Online. www.nap.edu/books/0309068371/html/. Accessed 12/3/05.

5. Leape, Lucian; Lawthers, Ann G.; Brennan, Troyen A., et al. (1993). Preventing Medical Injury. Qual Rev Bull. 19(5):144–149, 1993.

6. Berwick, D. (2000). Improving patient safety. Harvard Health Policy Review. Fall 2000; Volume 1, Number 1. Online. http://hcs.harvard.edu/~epihc/currentissue/fall2000/berwick.html

7. Berwick, D. (2000). Improving patient safety. Harvard Health Policy Review. Fall 2000; Volume 1, Number 1. Online. http://hcs.harvard.edu/~epihc/currentissue/fall2000/berwick.html

8. Orthostatic hypotension is the most common cardiovascular risk factor for falls, and the risk increases in persons over age 70. This problem involves a transient systolic blood pressure reduction of at least 20mmHg when the resident assumes an upright position. Volume depletion, bleeding, diarrhea, and certain medications commonly cause orthostasis, although many other factors may induce the

problem. The drop in blood pressure reduces blood flow to the brain, precipitating dizziness, loss of balance, or fainting that results in a fall. (Colgan J. Syncope: A fall from grace. Prog Cardiovasc Nurs. 2001;17(2):66-71.)

9. A toolkit of best practices for care of the elderly. Presentation. Ontario Hospital Association Conference. 2001. Online. www.joannabriggs.edu.au. Accessed 12/22/02.

10. Kuehm AF, Sendelweck S. Acute health status and its relationship to falls in the nursing home. J Gerontol Nurs. 1995;21(7):41-49.

11. American Nurses Association (ANA) standards of nursing practice require that documentation be based on the nursing process and that it should be ongoing and accessible to all members of the health care team. (Better Documentation. (1992). Springhouse, Pa.: Springhouse Corp., 39.)

12. Nursing encompasses the prevention of illness, the alleviation of suffering, and the protection, promotion, and restoration of health in the care of individuals, families, groups, and communities. Nurses act to change those aspects of social structures that detract from health and well-being. The Code for Nurses is the standard by which ethical conduct is guided and evaluated. It provides a framework within which nurses can make ethical decisions and discharge their professional responsibilities to the public, to other members of the health team, and to the profession. The Code for Nurses is not open to negotiation in employment settings, nor is it permissible for individuals, groups of nurses, or interested parties to adapt or change the language of this code. The Code for Nurses encompasses all nursing activities and may supersede specific policies of institutions, of employers, or of practices. Therefore, the content of the Code for Nurses with Interpretive Statements is nonnegotiable. Code for Nurses. (1985, 2001). Washington, D.C. American Nurses Publishing).

13. Oklahoma — You can't use the doc's apology against him. (2004). Nursing Home and Law Litigation Report. Vol. 4, No. 8. August 2004. Page 251.

14. The 'I'm sorry' movement is gaining momentum, unfortunately. (2004). Nursing Home and Law Litigation Report. Vol. 4, No. 8. August 2004. Page 251.

Quality assurance/benchmarking

The Director of Nursing (DON) in long-term care advocates for the assessment and evaluation of outcomes in the long-term care facility and develops implementation strategies for negative outcomes. The DON realizes the critical importance of Quality Assurance or any other type program which serves to seek out problems and strategize their solutions.[1]

The quality assessment and assurance committee

The Omnibus Budget Reconciliation (OBRA) regulations introduced long-term care facilities to a new requirement in the form of a mandate to establish a comprehensive quality assessment and assurance (QA & A) program. Our colleagues in hospitals and other branches of healthcare had been working under a similar mandate from the Joint Commission for at least 10 years. The current federal rules state:

F520 §483.75(o) Quality Assessment and Assurance

(1) A facility must maintain a quality assessment and assurance committee consisting of—
   (i) The director of nursing services;
   (ii) A physician designated by the facility; and
   (ii) At least three other members of the facility's staff.

The intent of this regulation is to ensure the facility has an established quality assurance committee that identifies and addresses quality issues and implements corrective action plans as necessary. Facility QA & A committees may be referred to by other names such as performance improvement or continuous quality Improvement committees but the functions and goals are the same. The quality assessment and assurance committee is responsible for identifying issues that necessitate action of the committee, such as issues that negatively affect quality of care and services provided to residents. In addition, the committee must develop and implement plans of action to correct identified deficiencies. The medical director may be the designated physician who serves on this committee.

Some facilities have been spared deficiencies because they were able to show that they had already identified and corrected problems through their QA program which were later identified by surveyors. The importance placed on quality assurance committees is seen in the *Guidelines to Surveyors* which state "If the facility has been out of compliance with a regulatory requirement between two surveys in which they were in compliance, that past noncompliance will not be cited by the survey team if a quality assurance program is in place and has corrected the noncompliance. An exception to this policy may be made in cases of egregious past noncompliance."

Almost every process reviewed by the QA & A committee can be explained in terms of four basic parameters: cost, time, customer (or employee) satisfaction, and errors or defects. Individual state rules have modified the original federal requirement for committee composition. In some states, facilities are required to expand their membership to include the facility administrator, a representative of the facility's governing body, and an individual who represents the residents. The frequency of the committee meetings may also be stipulated by individual state laws, but in most facilities the committee meets quarterly.

A commitment to quality

The keys to achieving quality are an organizational commitment, benchmarking data, and risk management. Promoting a culture of quality is helpful, but you must believe in it and commit to high quality care to be successful. Once you have committed to providing quality care, make quality improvement a priority.

Use the quality assurance committee to review incidents, pressure ulcers, restraints, catheters, infections, and other problem areas. However, do not limit the committee to these topics. Any potential problem may be reviewed. When evaluating incidents, pressure ulcers, and infections, remember to look at the big picture. Determine whether a dysfunction in the system caused the problem or set the stage for individual failure.

When evaluating quality, you must have a system for evaluating your activities and determining whether they have been successful. Facilities who emphasize teamwork, communication, and encourage direct-care staff involvement into resident plans of care are often success-ful with quality improvement efforts. These assets set the stage for quality care. Change is a constant in healthcare. Although there are many quality improvement models, the goals are essentially the same—to identify areas in which change is needed and implement changes to improve processes of care delivery.

You may want to develop checklists for doing quality review audits. List the current standards of care for the area you are evaluating. Review the state and federal rules and make sure to include all the requirements. In some situations, record review may provide all the information you need to determine whether services are delivered effectively. In others, you must do direct observation on the units, and interview staff and residents or responsible parties. Much will depend on the subject you are studying. When auditing for quality, try to think of all related factors and do not leave any stones unturned. You will find an example audit and a blank tem-plate form on the CD-ROM that accompanies your book.

In 2002, CMS took quality improvement one step beyond the QA & A Committee when they introduced the quality measures. In 2004, a set of advanced quality measures was released. Quality indicators (QI) (also called quality measures QM) are identified by using data on the MDS assessments. MDS data are transmitted to the state long-term care survey office, then sent to the federal government. The government collects information concerning the resi-dents' physical and clinical conditions and abilities, preferences, and life care wishes.

After the assessment data are converted into quality measures, they are posted on the Medi-care Web page so they can be used as a source of information with which to evaluate facility services. When facilities consider "reportable events" they often think of abuse, neglect and misappropriation of property. In reality, because of the MDS system, every fall, weight loss, pressure ulcer and numerous other data are reported to the state through the MDS submis-sion process. Most of the quality measures reflect a resident's condition for the seven days before the MDS was completed, so they may not represent the resident's condition accurately. For example, residents were assessed for pain over the past seven days. Pain that was subse-quently relieved will not be reflected until the assessment is updated. Because of this, facilities should have mechanisms to monitor current data on an ongoing basis.

Monitoring quality indicators has become popular in healthcare. Quality indicators are a benchmark of sorts. There are many free tools for research and decision-making available online. These can be used for identifying and recognizing potential problem areas, tracking changes in performance and outcomes, and identifying areas that need further study and re-search. Indicators that reflect facility services can be measured. Since facilities are required to have systems in place for recording and reviewing events such as falls, skin tears, med errors etc., they should put these data to work as a part of their QA program. This develops the facility's own benchmarks and a basis upon which to initiate improvement. How many falls did you have last month, last year? Are you utilizing the data to develop a culture of safety awareness in your facility? Stepping from reactive to proactive involves incorporating the information from risk assessments into the QA process. Instead of waiting for a resident to fall and developing an intervention, you act upon the risk assessment to prevent the fall in the first place.

The quality measures used by CMS were selected because the issues are important to resident care. All of the QI's reflect conditions that can be modified or corrected, so facilities have a means of changing and/or improving their scores. Comparing the indicators also provides a means of comparing your facility and its residents with other facilities. They provide a snapshot of how facilities and their residents are different from one another, and how they are alike.

The online quality measures have been validated and are research-based. Statistical methods have been applied to adjust measures that are out of a facility's control, so as not to lower the score unfairly. The quality measures are posted on the Nursing Home Compare Web site at *www.medicare.gov* so that any interested person can access the data. Facilities are encouraged to check the information posted on the web site. If you find errors in your facility's data, inform CMS of the problem and ask them to correct it.

Benchmarking

Benchmarking is part of the quality improvement process. A benchmark is a standard reference point against which performance is measured. Benchmarking is an activity in which a facility establishes "best practices" by comparing what they are doing with similar facilities. The supply of data that can be benchmarked is limitless. Any aspect of the organization can be benchmarked. To make a comparison, you must be familiar with the standard of care for the clinical area being compared. If you are unsure of the current standards, benchmarking is helpful in identifying the applicable standard of care. By benchmarking with other organizations, the facility can improve its processes and achieve excellence.

Critical thinking is an essential skill for quality assurance. It is used for problem solving, brainstorming potential solutions, drawing conclusions, combining information, separating fact from opinion, or identifying potential outcomes. Benchmarking involves applying critical thinking to learn what other facilities are doing, and using the information to solve problems in your own facility. This does not involve copying what others are doing. Once a problem has been identified, you apply practices that are likely to work. This may mean employing many approaches from several different facilities, and modifying them to fit your situation.

Root cause analysis

Root cause analysis (RCA) is used for identifying the cause or contributing factors associated with untoward events. It employs critical thinking to identify solutions to problems. Your facility will have guidelines for conducting a root cause analysis investigation. Root cause analyses:

- Should involve an interdisciplinary team, making sure that personnel are knowledgeable about the processes involved

- Emphasizes systems and processes rather than individual performance

- Focuses on determining what happened and why it happened; it asks questions repeatedly until all aspects of the process are reviewed and contributing factors identified

- Makes recommendations for procedural changes to reduce the risk of untoward events and incidents

After the root cause analysis is done, the team will write a root cause statement. The root cause statement:

- Identifies the cause and effect of the incident or event being studied.

- Answers all obvious questions.

- Operates on the premise that most incidents have multiple potential underlying causes; there is seldom only one cause of an untoward event.

- Avoids negative terminology; uses only positive terms.

- Recognizes that each human error has a cause. Procedure violations are usually not considered root causes. Each violation must have a preceding cause. Failure to act is only a root cause if the staff member has a duty to act.

- Determines whether workplace or system redesign will reduce the risk of incident recurrence.

- Is consistent and not contradictory.

- Considers relevant literature and standards.

- Includes recommendations for corrective actions and outcome measures.

Root cause analysis focuses on learning how an incident occurred. It is not a punitive process and does not place blame. The team uses what they have learned to make recommendations for preventive measures and solutions. Transparency is essential to root cause analysis. This means the information is available to others. The results of an investigation are not useful unless they are accessible and understandable. Facility staff and interested others should know how and where to access the information.

Lack of root cause analysis opened the door to a dozen lawsuits for one hospital. Newborn infants and one mother spontaneously developed respiratory distress as a result of surreptitious Lidocaine injections by a technician. The United States District Court for the Middle District of Alabama scrutinized the incident reports and other documentation in great detail. The jurists determined there was an obvious pattern to the incidents. The presence of a pattern should have caused the hospital to investigate to determine whether the incidents were random or isolated, or if a pattern of personnel or other circumstances existed.

The court ruled the hospital had a legal responsibility to identify and eliminate the cause of the problem long before a dozen patients were injured. The court stated that one purpose of quality assurance is to be aware of the possibility of suspicious patterns in adverse episodes. If a potential pattern of ongoing intentional criminal misconduct exists, the QA committee must take steps to identify it. A good place to start is matching up the personnel on duty with the incidents, then reviewing and/or investigating their backgrounds. The court noted that a hospital can be liable for negligence if patients continue to be harmed after events have provided an opportunity for the QA committee to notice the problem and act on it.[2]

Customer and employee satisfaction

In addition to improving quality of care, some facilities are reviewing consumer satisfaction and have borrowed ideas from the retail industry to ensure the residents and families are happy. Staff turnover reduction is also an area of intense study. Facilities realize that turnover is expensive, so the quality assurance program studies and implements new methods for employee satisfaction and staff retention.

Best practices

Best practices are procedures, programs, or activities that are successful and can be readily adopted by other individuals or organizations. These practices may be considered leading edge, or exceptional models for others to follow. Many facilities share best practices that have been effective and have been successful in improving some aspect of facility life or services. Several states and quality improvement organizations post this information on their Web pages for others to download. Many tools are available to help you evaluate care. You may wish to check your state nursing facility regulatory web page, state health department, and any of the many best practice and quality information Web sites.

The governing body

The governing body or board of directors has been named as a party to many lawsuits. The generally low reimbursement rate, intensive regulatory scrutiny, and overall demands of facility operations have made it difficult for the individual or family-owned facilities to survive. Most facilities have corporate ownership. Plaintiffs often allege that the corporate approach has reduced the quality of care. However, without the corporately-owned facility some communities would not have long-term care services available.

Plaintiffs commonly allege corporate greed. Sympathetic juries have awarded millions in punitive damages to send the corporate owners a message. Without taking a position in this argument, facilities must be aware that the governing body has a responsibility for quality, and thus they have a stake in the activities of the QA & A committee. The QA & A committee should have some means of communicating with and reporting their activities to the governing body.

The requirements for the governing body are interspersed with information about survey compliance, as well as billing fraud and abuse. However, the governing body clearly also bears a responsibility for regulatory compliance and quality of care. In a document providing guidance to members of the governing body, the General Accounting Office (GAO) summarizes the responsibilities of the facility directors.[3] The governing body's responsibilities include determining the mission, goals and objectives of the facility. These important functions set the tone for quality care.

The facility must have policies, procedures, and written standards of conduct and professional services that have been endorsed by the governing body. The standards should be binding on all employees and other professionals, independent contractors, and volunteers performing services for the nursing facility, as well as other providers operating under the nursing facility's control, such as therapy companies, durable medical equipment suppliers and laboratories. The code of conduct describes the facility's commitment to ethical behavior, and identifies expectations of employees. The code should also make a commitment to legal compliance. It helps define the facility's culture by detailing the fundamental principles, values, and framework for action within the facility. You would expect the general operating policies to derive from its principles. The code represents the facility's ethical philosophy, and the policies and procedures represent the organization's response and methods of managing the daily operations and problems the facility confronts.

The code of conduct should be implemented by written policies and procedures that facility staff should follow. The compliance officer is usually assisted by the QA & A committee, who analyze problems and advises on strategies for improvement and promoting regulatory compliance. The board of directors should satisfy itself that management has developed a system that establishes accountability for proper implementation of the compliance program.

The GAO notes that the experience of many organizations is that program implementation lags where there is poor distribution of responsibility, authority and accountability beyond the compliance officer. They note that facilities must act on deficiencies or suspected noncompliance promptly. Failure to respond to a known deficiency may be considered an aggravating circumstance in evaluating the organization's potential liability for the underlying problem. In addition, the Board should receive sufficient information to evaluate the appropriateness of the organization's response.[4] Since the governing body is often the legal entity licensed by the state to operate the facility, final responsibility for facility operations rests with this body. This body must be kept informed of quality assurance activities and approve changes in operating policies and procedures.

Confidentiality of QA & A committee data

Surveyors are expected to question facility staff and review documents only for the purpose of determining whether the facility has a quality assurance committee, and whether the committee is used for the intended purpose of identifying and addressing problematic (or potentially problematic) issues. Surveyors are not to use QA committee minutes or findings as a basis for writing deficiencies. The rules imply that the QA data are protected and need not be disclosed: §483.75(o) (3) A State or the Secretary may not require disclosure of the records of such committee except insofar as such disclosure is related to the compliance of such committee with the requirements of this section. (4) Good faith attempts by the committee to identify and correct quality deficiencies will not be used as a basis for sanctions.

Because of this rule, facilities tend to place a great deal of potentially damaging information under the auspices of the QA & A committee. For example, they consider all investigations of alleged abuse and neglect, incident reports, information about in-house pressure ulcer development, and nosocomial infections to be protected quality assurance information that is not disclosed to surveyors, or anyone else. The protected information privilege has been the subject of a number of court rulings in many states. In many rulings, the various courts have required facilities to release the information they considered protected. Court opinions from one state are not necessarily limited to the state of origin. If a similar issue comes before the court in any state, documents and opinions on related subjects from other states are likely to be reviewed and considered. Court opinions are often lengthy and copying them is beyond the scope of this book. However, relevant parts are snipped from several court rulings. The source document can be readily accessed for additional, more comprehensive information.

"The Legislature recognized the chilling effect that would be engendered by enfeebling confidentiality. . . . We agree that, "[o]nce a state has made the policy decision to afford privileged status for certain records, the Legislature and the courts should not undermine the policy objective by circumventing or weakening the privileged status with exceptions not mandated by constitutional considerations or the long-term interests of justice. Nothing is worse than a halfhearted privilege; it becomes a game of semantics that leaves parties twisting in the wind while lawyers determine its scope." (Quoting Charles David Creech, The Medical Review Committee Privilege: A Jurisdictional Survey, 67 N.C.L. Rev. 179, 179-80 (1988))."

"Texas courts have not carved out new exceptions to the peer-review committee privilege but have simply applied the peer-review privilege to prevent what the appellant now attempts to do—namely, cloak public information in confidentiality by first filtering it through the peer-review process. In Irving, the court limited the privilege to those documents created by the committee itself. Texas courts have consistently limited the peer-review committee privileges to those documents generated by the committee as a result of the committee's deliberative processes and to those submitted to the committee at their direction and in furtherance of committee business. See Memorial Hosp.—The Woodlands v. McCown, 927 S.W.2d 1, 9 (Tex. 1996); Barnes v. Whittington, 751 S.W.2d 493, 496 (Tex. 1988); Jordan v. Court of Appeals, 701 S.W.2d 644, 647-48 (Tex. 1985); Texarkana Mem'l Hosp., Inc. v. Jones, 551 S.W.2d 33, 34-36 (Tex. 1977); Ebony Lake, 62 S.W.3d at 869; see also Creech, supra at 184 (noting that the privilege is limited to what the committee produces). Just because a report may deal with a nursing home's quality of care and has been reviewed by a peer-review committee does not necessarily mean that the report is cloaked with a committee privilege." (Capital Senior Management 1, Inc. v. Texas Department of Human Services 03-02-00615-CV [Tex.App. Dist.3 03/11/2004])

In a lawsuit against a long-term care facility, the plaintiffs filed a writ to compel the facility to release their surveys. The appeals court addressed the issue of whether a long-term care facility investigation report prepared by the state survey agency, the facility's plans of correction, and the testimony of surveyors regarding their investigations are excluded from lawsuit discovery under the peer review privilege. The plaintiff asked the appellate court to order the trial court to permit use of the survey reports during discovery and at trial. The facility resisted, claiming peer review privilege.

They argued that the surveyors' reports were prepared from confidential information that the facility's peer review committee provided. (This is not necessarily true, because the surveyors reviewed resident records and data that may also have been reviewed by the QA & A committee.) As a result, they contended the information was privileged and should not be released. The facility stated that surveys were part of the peer review process. (In this facility, the QA & A committee also reviewed survey findings.) The court noted that there was no evidence that the survey reports disclosed any confidential information. The opinion stated that the mere fact that the facility's peer review committee may have reviewed the documents did not make them privileged.

The Court of Appeals noted that the civil statutes that protect the peer review privilege do not apply when records are required or authorized by law to be disclosed. In this case, surveys and plans of correction must be posted in the facility and are considered a public record. The court determined that the peer review privilege extends to documents prepared by or at the direction of a peer review committee for committee purposes. Other documents, such as surveys that are submitted to a committee or that are created without committee impetus and purpose are not protected. (In re Donna Pack, 996 S.W.2d 4 [Tex. App.—Fort Worth 1999 n.w.h.])

"Identifying opportunities for change generally represents a departure from traditional patterns and methods of doing business. Examining the purpose of health care and re-directing commitments toward new goals, demands strong partnerships, not only internally, but externally with the community. A well conceived and developed planning process can build and strengthen these alliances."

The State Supreme Court opinions

Supreme court opinions are also quite lengthy. The Texas court system has also addressed the confidentiality of records and peer-reviewed documents at many levels, and their decisions provide helpful information and guidance on this issue. The Supreme Court of Texas heard a case in 2004 in which the facility had filed a Writ of Mandamus. This is an extraordinary action that is used to command an official to perform an act as an absolute duty that is not left to the individual's discretion.

A writ of mandamus action is typically used only when all other judicial remedies have failed. In Texas, a person may obtain mandamus relief only if (1) the trial court clearly abused its discretion and (2) the party requesting mandamus has no adequate remedy by appeal. In this case, the trial court had previously ordered the facility to produce documents that lacked a

"QA & A privilege" stamp, and privilege log documents that did not have the word "committee" in the name to the plaintiff.

The issue reviewed on appeal was brought by a long-term care facility that was being sued for wrongful death and providing negligent care. After being served with discovery, the facility withheld many internal documents, asserting the medical peer review privilege and the quality assessment and assurance privilege. The plaintiff filed a motion to compel (demand) production of the documents. The facility was required to submit various documents for judicial review, including an affidavit from the director of nursing.

An affidavit is a formal sworn statement or written declaration made under oath. It is witnessed, usually by a notary public or other person who is legally authorized to administer an oath. The affidavit described the QA & A committee activities and explained that the privileged documents were logged. The documents submitted for review were of two types:

1. Information and reports prepared for the committees to review

2. Reports generated by the committee

The facility's QA & A plan stated that documents prepared or reviewed by the QA & A committee will be stamped with a confidentiality statement that reads, "This report has been generated as part of the facility's quality assessment and assurance process and constitutes confidential Quality Assessment and Assurance Committee records." However, not all the documents submitted for judicial review were stamped.

The QA & A plan noted that four privileges were protected by the peer review process under the auspices of the quality assurance committee. These were the:

- Medical committee privilege

- Medical peer review committee privilege

- Nursing peer review committee privilege

- Quality assessment and assurance privilege

In deciding this case,[5] the Supreme Court of Texas referred to several previous opinions, which stated that both "the medical committee privilege and the medical peer review privilege extended to initial credentialing by medical committees." It also applied to other confidential documents that are "generated" by a committee or "prepared by or at the direction of the committee for committee purposes." Privileged documents included the "minutes and recommendations" of medical committees, inquiries about a physician to other sources and the sources' responses, and communications between the physician and the facility. They added that "simply passing a document through a peer review committee does not make it privileged."

In the previous opinions, the justices noted that the statutes did not protect documents that were "made or maintained in the regular course of business by a hospital or extended care facility." They interpreted this to mean that medical records should be evaluated to determine whether they were made "in the regular course of business." Business records excepted from the peer review privilege include a "patient's medical records" and "business and administrative files and papers apart from committee deliberations." The justices noted that the QA & A committee was authorized to evaluate the quality of healthcare services, so it was comparable or similar to a medical peer review committee. As a medical committee, QA & A committee documents are privileged, except as limited by the business records exception.

The Texas Occupations Code[6] is a legal statute that defines regulated occupations, such as physicians and nurses, in which state licensure or registration is required. The justices previously ruled that a medical peer review committee has the authority "to evaluate the quality of medical and health care services, such as the administration of drugs by a nurse at the instruction of a physician." They noted, "The purpose of medical peer review is protection of an evaluative process, not mere recordkeeping."

A nursing peer review committee is also defined by the Occupations Code.[7] The justices noted that, "Separate from the medical committee and the medical peer review committee, a "nursing peer review committee" is the entity authorized to engage in nurse peer review." To qualify as a nursing peer review committee, nurses must comprise at least three-fourths of the membership of the committee. Thus, the long-term care facility may only assert the nursing peer review privilege if the committee meets the narrow and rigorous membership requirements defined in the occupations code.

Since the facility's QA & A plan defined its nursing peer review committee as consisting of the Administrator, Director of Nursing, Medical Director or other designated physician, social service representative, dietary representative, and a Certified Nursing Assistant, it did not meet this definition. The facility did not submit proof that three-fourths of the membership consisted of nurses. Because of this, the justices ruled that the nursing peer review privilege did not apply in this case.

Although the facility clearly won some concessions, the justices ruled that many of the documents at issue in this case fell outside the range of documents protected by the medical committee and medical peer review privileges. The documents withheld by the facility included surveys and documents that concern licensing and investigation by state agencies. Records included information about employees, as well as incident logs and other reports referencing the plaintiff.

Additional documents withheld by the facility included governing body meeting minutes, personnel records including documentation of training, and policy and procedure documents. The judicial opinion noted that, "The peer review privilege is intended to extend far enough to foster candid internal discussions for the purpose of making improvements in the quality of care, but not so far as to permit the concealment of 'routinely accumulated information.' "[T]he privilege [does] not prevent discovery of material that ha[s] been presented to a committee if it [is] otherwise available and 'offered or proved by means apart from the record of the committee." The privilege extends only to the products of the peer review process: reports, records (including those produced for the committee's review as part of the investigative review process), and deliberations.

The plaintiff in this case alleged that the facility waived its claim of privilege by failing to follow its own policies because it had not stamped the documents with a QA & A privilege statement. The court disagreed, noting that under the current rules of discovery, inadvertent disclosure does not automatically waive a claim of privilege. Similarly, they held that a party's inadvertent failure to utilize its own internal procedure for identifying privileged documents does not automatically waive the privilege. They noted, however, that the absence of the confidentiality stamp may also be relevant, so the trial court would not abuse its discretion by weighing the lack of stamp, in addition to considering the reason for its absence, along with the DON's affidavit, the QA & A privilege log, and the sample documents, in determining whether the facility met its burden to demonstrate that the documents at issue were part of the peer review process.

They noted further in camera review should be done by the trial court. An in camera review is done by submitting the documents in question to the judge, who will review them privately. The information is not made public or submitted to the jury until the judge has rendered a decision on its admissibility. Of all the sample documents submitted in this case, the Supreme Court of Texas noted that the only ones that may possibly be privileged were the "Incident Report QA & A logs" and the "Weekly Pressure Ulcer QA & A logs." The trial court had previously limited its in camera review to only those documents that were stamped with the QA & A committee stamp, and these had not been stamped.

The justices noted that further review of the documents was needed, and left the final determination of privilege for the sample Incident Report logs and Weekly Pressure Ulcer logs to the trial court. All other documents submitted were determined to be clearly outside the privilege because:

- They do not pertain exclusively to physicians;

- They pertain to nurses, but the facility did not establish a nurse peer review committee consistent with the statutory requirement; or

- They were contemporaneous resident records made in the ordinary course of business and were not specifically created for committee review, evaluation, or investigation.

The court opinion noted that "the trial court considered only the name of the documents or whether the documents were stamped with the QA & A indicia, and failed to consider other determining factors, including the purpose for which the documents were created. The trial court must determine:

- Whether the existing evidence establishes the privileged status of any documents without the need for an in camera inspection;

- Whether to conduct an in camera inspection of additional documents or categories of documents in light of this opinion;

- Whether the additional documents, if furnished, are privileged; and

- Whether the long-term care facility, by failing to produce all documents for in camera inspection, failed to satisfy its burden to prove privilege.

They concluded that the facility was entitled to mandamus relief because the trial court abused its discretion by using only superficial indicators to deny the facility's privilege claim as to nearly all the documents at issue. They directed the trial court to vacate its original discovery order and determine whether, upon further examination, any documents withheld by the facility may be considered privileged.[8]

This is a complex opinion that draws on many other judicial opinions, but the implications for facilities in every state are clear:

- Simply passing a document through a peer review (QA & A) committee does not make it privileged.

- Recordkeeping of meetings and committee business should be precise enough to determine what type of information is being reviewed, deficiencies identified, and action or recommendations taken as a result of this review.

- If numerous documents, such as incident reports are reviewed, some type of log should be maintained with committee records.

- Facilities should follow their policies and procedures regarding maintaining QA & A committee logs and stamping items as confidential.

- Facilities should learn if their state has legal definitions of peer review, nursing peer review, and other committees and determine whether their in-house committees function according to the legal definitions. If not, the privilege protections may not apply.

- Facilities should learn whether peer review protections in their state apply only to organizations such as hospitals, physician practices, and others. The law should specify whether long-term care facilities are also afforded peer review protection.

- Facilities should learn if the state law exempts any documents from peer review privilege, and if so, how these exceptions apply.

Effective quality assurance

Do not allow the legalities of disclosure or immunity of information to alter your plan for quality assurance. Effective quality assurance programs may be your best investment into avoiding lawsuits in the first place. A team approach and root cause analysis can reduce pressure ulcers, falls, psychoactive medications, weight loss and a myriad of other issues often cited as the basis for lawsuits. In the end an effective quality assurance program may well be your best defense and your resident's best friend.

References

1. National Association of Directors of Nursing Administration/Long Term Care (NADONA) (eds). (2000). Standards of Practice (4th edition). Cincinnati, OH. National Association of Directors of Nursing Administration/Long Term Care.

2. Gess vs. U.S., 952 F. Supp. 1529 (M.D. Ala., 1996).

3. Office of Inspector General and American Health Lawyers Association (Eds.). (2003). Corporate responsibility and corporate compliance: a resource for health care boards of directors. Rockville, MD. U.S. Department of Health and Human Services. Online. http://oig.hhs.gov/fraud/docs/complianceguidance/040203CorpRespRsceGuide.pdf. Accessed 01/20/06.

4. Office of Inspector General and American Health Lawyers Association (Eds.). (2003). Corporate responsibility and corporate compliance: a resource for health care boards of directors. Rock-

ville, MD. U.S. Department of Health and Human Services. Online. http://oig.hhs.gov/fraud/docs/complianceguidance/040203CorpRespRsceGuide.pdf. Accessed 01/20/06.

5. In Re Living Centers of Texas, Inc., D/B/A Wharton Manor, Relator. No. 04-0176. In the Supreme Court of Texas. October 14, 2005.

6. Texas Statutes. Occupations Code. Online. www.capitol.state.tx.us/statutes/octoc.html.

7. "Nursing peer review committee" means a committee established under the authority of the governing body of a national, state, or local nursing association, a school of nursing, the nursing staff of a hospital, health science center, nursing home, home health agency, temporary nursing service, or other health care facility, or state agency or political subdivision for the purpose of conducting peer review. The committee includes an employee or agent of the committee, including an assistant, an investigator, an intervenor, an attorney, and any other person who serves the committee in any capacity. (5) "Peer review" means the evaluation of nursing services, the qualifications of a nurse, the quality of patient care rendered by a nurse, the merits of a complaint concerning a nurse or nursing care, and a determination or recommendation regarding a complaint. The term includes: (A) the evaluation of the accuracy of a nursing assessment and observation and the appropriateness and quality of the care rendered by a nurse; (B) a report made to a nursing peer review committee concerning an activity under the committee's review authority; (C) a report made by a nursing peer review committee to another committee or to the board as permitted or required by law; and (D) implementation of a duty of a nursing peer review committee by a member, an agent, or an employee of the committee. (Acts 1999, 76th Leg., ch. 388, § 1, eff. Sept. 1, 1999. Amended by Acts 2003, 78th Leg., ch. 553, § 2.018, eff. Feb. 1, 2004.)

8. In Re Living Centers of Texas, Inc., D/B/A Wharton Manor, Relator. No. 04-0176. In the Supreme Court of Texas. October 14, 2005.

9. Zagury CS. Making a difference: Strategic planning for the director of nursing in long term care. The Director. Online. www.nadona.org/media_archive/media/media-238.pdf. Accessed 08/25/04.

Documentation

A complete medical record reflects the documentation of high-quality, nonnegligent care and is your best defense against allegations of negligence. It should reflect an accurate and complete account of the care rendered. Let's compare a complete and accurate medical record to a book: It's a story of this patient's care at this point in his or her life. It should have a beginning, middle, and an end.

When reading a medical record, any reviewer should get a good clinical picture of the events, care, and outcome of the patient. There should be no incomplete flow sheets, incomplete graphic sheets, or lapses in progress notes. All notes should include the correct date, time, and accounting of the clinical status, as well as the clinical care provided. Many times, when reviewing a clinical record, these simple items—date and time of assessment—are missing. Although they may seem inconsequential to the nurse, date and time can be used to demonstrate critical missing care at a critical time.

Risk management recommendations to give staff

To ensure well-documented resident records, consider using some of these risk-management guidelines:

- Document all care given. This documentation will be measured by your state's Nurse Practice Act and standards of professional nursing practice. It also serves as proof that care was, in fact, given. Document conversations with providers. Include highlights of the conversation, date and time of the conversation, and the provider's response, instructions, and orders.

- Document the nursing interventions that occurred before and after notifying the provider.

- If the chain of command was used, document who was contacted, the time of the call, the message communicated, and the response to it.

- Always complete all forms/documentation tools.

- Document all sponge counts (e.g., in the operating room, in labor and delivery).

- Document what instructions the patient was given as well as any conversations with the patient/family.

- Use only the accepted methods for correcting chart errors in the medical record.

- Do not document opinions.

- Never blame another individual or department in the clinical record.

Help your staff document

In addition to physicians' documentation, nurses' (and therapists') documentation affects patient safety, reimbursement, risk management, and more, so it's important that everyone work to keep thorough and accurate documentation. The following pointers can help your nursing staff improve their documentation:

- **Train immediately**—The time of hire is a good time to explain the expectations for documentation and the legal ramifications of inadequate documentation. In some facilities, new nurses go through an orientation and are buddied up with another RN, who goes through nurses' notes, assessment, daily care records, and medication records.

- **Provide ongoing feedback**—Use case studies for annual updates. It's also useful to provide feedback after documentation to be sure that nurses change the way they document when necessary. In addition to an annual program, some hospitals discuss documentation problems during staff meetings or quarterly nursing-rounds case studies.

- **Focus on legibility**—Health Information Management (HIM) could select charts, block out names, and show as examples documentation with critical elements (for either quality issues or reimbursement issues) missing or impossible to read. People are likely to realize their handwriting is illegible.

- **Develop useful forms**—Reduce redundancy. Work closely with staff to develop flow sheets that would meet nurses' needs as well as those of the Joint Commission and other regulators. Monitor success through chart auditing.

- **Work toward computerization**—Move toward a computerized record system that leads the user to complete, timely, and accurate documentation. It also eliminates problems with illegible entries and gaps in documentation, and it captures critical clinical data for use in case review, benchmarking for quality, and reimbursement.

In today's lawsuit-laden society, nurse managers need to understand that the clinical record can either avert a potential lawsuit or provide credibility to plaintiff allegations that the care provided was negligent. The clinical record is the only document that will demonstrate whether all of the care rendered by everyone on the healthcare team was up to the standard level of care.

Understand that although documentation seems burdensome and not the top priority of a busy day, it will be your salvation if the patient/family believes that care did not meet their expectations. This is especially true when a patient files or voices a complaint about his or her care or when there is an adverse medical event, such as a fall or medication error.

Documentation standards

Most lawsuits involving long-term care facilities and their nurses are civil cases that attempt to prove that negligent nursing care resulted in injury to a resident. Negligence is failure to provide a resident with the standard of care that a reasonably prudent nurse would exercise under the same or similar circumstances. To prove that a nurse (or facility) was negligent, the resident's attorney must prove these four elements:

- The nurse (or facility) had a duty to provide care to the resident and to follow an acceptable standard of care.

- The nurse (or facility) failed to adhere to the standard of care.

- The nurse's (or facility's) failure to adhere to the standard of care caused the resident's injuries.

- The resident suffered damages as a result of the nurse's (or facility's) negligent actions.

The professional practice standard for long-term care requires nursing facilities to maintain clinical records for each resident, in accordance with accepted professional health information management standards and practices, that are complete; accurately documented; readily accessible; and systematically organized. Jurors often expect healthcare professionals to be above reproach. Think about it. Healthcare workers are entrusted with peoples' lives. They make life-and-death decisions.

When a case goes before a jury, jurors generally expect documentation to be factual and honest. As you can see, documentation can be very important when an individual or facility are facing allegations of negligence. Naturally, all parties involved will contend that they provided care that met the applicable standard, and that it is always their practice to do so. This position may be markedly weakened if documentation does not reflect that the applicable standards were met. During a trial, expect the plaintiff's attorney to use the medical record to prove that the standard of care was not met.

In healthcare, there is a maxim, "If it's not charted, it wasn't done." Although what is written in the medical records could harm you in court, omissions can make the damage seem insurmountable. Without proper documentation, a reader may assume that no care was provided. Although some facilities use a system called "charting by exception," most adhere to the age-old maxim and chart all care given. Charting by exception (CBE) is a formal documentation system. It has formal, written policies and procedures and well-designed flow sheets and forms. It is not an excuse for haphazard charting.

Even in a charting-by-exception system, the state nurse practice act always prevails. Most states have a clause similar to this one: "The nurse shall accurately and completely report and document the client's status including signs, symptoms and responses; nursing care rendered; physician, dentist or podiatrist orders; administration of medications, and treatments; and client response(s); contacts with other healthcare team members concerning significant events regarding client's status."[1] Thus, even in a charting-by-exception system, the nurse must have a means of documenting care given and the resident's response, as well as the other elements listed above.

Documentation is a critical part of nursing practice, not an afterthought. Some nurses say, "The residents come first; paperwork is secondary." This is probably a good practice to ascribe to, assuming that the paperwork is completed after residents are cared for. Omitting paperwork entirely is never a good practice. American Nurses Association (ANA) standards of nursing practice require that documentation be based on the nursing process and that it should be ongoing and accessible to all members of the healthcare team.[2] View documentation as an important part of the care you give. A medical-legal chart reviewer will be able to identify the various aspects of the nursing process during a documentation review. The purpose of documentation is to communicate care. Documentation is a true, complete, objective record of the care given and the residents' response. It is the first line of defense in proving accountability.

The long-term care nursing facility must maintain clinical records on each resident, in accordance with accepted professional health information management standards and practices, that are complete; accurately documented; readily accessible; and systematically organized. It is my opinion that the EFG Care Center records were negligently kept or the records were deliberately scrambled and disorganized prior to my receiving them. The record was in a mess as far as its organization; it was not provided in the same manner as usually kept in the ordinary course of business. It did not meet the standard for closed records. As stated previously, some photocopies were illegible, and many parts appear to have been redacted.

If a facility and/or its personnel are sued, all verbal testimony will be considered, contrasted, and compared with documentation on the medical record. The nurses can testify that their normal practice is to turn residents every two hours and provide other preventive skin care. However, the jury is not obligated to believe this testimony, especially if the medical record does not show evidence of regular turning and repositioning.

In this case, documentation skips most probably support the injuries that the resident and/or family are alleging. This situation occurred in a 2004 lawsuit against a Kentucky hospital. The family filed suit for nursing negligence based on a patient who fell and sustained a fracture, then subsequently developed a Stage III pressure ulcer. Her condition deteriorated to the point where the healthcare proxy decided to withhold her regular dialysis treatments and the patient died. Despite verbal nursing testimony, documentation on the medical record was erratic, inconsistent, and did not show evidence of routine turning or preventive skin care. When skin breakdown became evident, a wound care nurse consultation was ordered, but the nurse did not respond in a timely manner. The physician ordered a special pressure-relieving bed. Nurses' notes confirmed the bed was not provided for more than 48 hours after the order was written. The jury did not believe the nurses' testimony about routine preventive skin care in light of the erratic documentation and delays in consultation and special pressure-relieving equipment. They found in favor of the plaintiff, and the Court of Appeals upheld the jury verdict.[3]

Requirements for nursing documentation

American Nurses Association standards of nursing practice require that documentation be based on the nursing process and that it should be ongoing and accessible to all members of the healthcare team.[4] Nursing documentation should be:

- Based upon the requirements of your state's Nurse Practice Act

- Objective—not critical or subjective

- Clear, concise and comprehensive

- Accurate, truthful, and honest—does not appear self-serving, especially if an incident or injury occurs

- Relevant and appropriate

- Reflective of observations, not of unfounded conclusions

- Reflective of resident education

- Reflective of resident response to care and actions taken to rectify unsatisfactory response

- Timely and completed only during or after giving care

- Chronological

- Internally consistent

- A complete record of nursing care provided, including assessments, identification of health issues, a plan of care, implementation and evaluation

- Legible and nonerasable

- Unaltered

- Permanent

- Retrievable

- Confidential

- Resident-focused

- Outcome-based

- Completed using forms, methods, systems provided or methods and systems consistent with these standards, facility policies, and state laws

Confidentiality of medical records and identifiable resident information

As you know, each resident has a right to privacy with regard to his or her medical information. The residents' medical records are always privileged and confidential documents. All staff are responsible for protecting resident information and data from access by unauthorized persons. Medical records and other resident data should be accessed only by those with a need to know the information. Staff should not be permitted to read resident charts out of curiosity.

In 1996, congress passed the Health Insurance Portability and Accountability Act (HIPAA). This law has many provisions. Protected health information (PHI) is the nucleus of the HIPAA privacy regulations. The purpose of the HIPAA rules is to:

- Increase resident control over their medical records

- Restrict the use and disclosure of resident information (however, residents cannot refuse to permit state and federal access to electronically-transmitted resident assessment instrument information)

- Make facilities accountable for protecting resident data

- Require the facility to implement and monitor the effectiveness of their information-release policies and procedures

The HIPAA rules ask providers to analyze how and where resident information is used, and develop procedures for protecting confidential data. This includes the areas where resident charts are stored, the places where private or identifying resident information is discussed, and how residents' personal health information is distributed. The HIPAA policies and procedures are written by and individualized to the facility.

The HIPAA regulations describe:

- What information is considered PHI

- The circumstances in which PHI may be disclosed

- The rights of an individual who is the subject of the PHI

Under the HIPAA rules, residents have the right to:

- Know about uses and disclosure of their own PHI

- Inspect their medical records

- Decide whether their PHI can be disclosed and to whom

- Correct inaccurate information in their medical records

Anything that potentially reveals the resident's identity is PHI. This includes:

- Names on a roster posted on the wall or by the doorway to the room (unless the resident consents)

- Lists (such as supplement lists, restraint lists, BM lists, etc.) posted at the nurses' station in public view

- Photographs of residents (unless the resident consents)

- Admission and discharge data

Since the HIPAA regulations protect all individually identifiable health information in any form, the rules apply to paper, verbal, and electronic documentation, billing records, and medical or clinical records. They cover virtually all communications made by the long-term care facility. Resident information is provided to staff on a "need to know" basis.

The premise of this requirement is that information is disclosed only if staff need it to carry out their duties. For example, the dietary department would need to know if a resident was on a diabetic diet. They would not need to know that the resident has an infectious disease. The nursing staff would need to know about both the diabetes and the infection. The MDS nurse may need to read the entire chart to complete the RAI.

However, other employees such as the pharmacist, dietitian, nursing assistant, social worker, activities, and others should be given access to limited areas of the medical record. Vendors should not be given free access to resident charts because of the potential for Medicare and Medicaid fraud. The facility should not allow access to a resident's clinical record unless a physician's order exists for supplies, equipment, or services provided by the entity seeking access to the record. Facilities must monitor how and where they use resident information. Policies must protect resident charts, conversations and reports about resident information, faxing resident documents, emailing or using a wireless transmitter to send electronic information, and disclosing other personal information.

Examples of violation of the HIPAA rules are:

- Disclosing personal resident details on computer monitors facing public areas

- Discussing residents in areas in which conversations can be overheard

- Misdirecting mail

- Discarding PHI in the regular trash without shredding

- Discarding feeding tube, catheter, or IV bags with resident names in the regular trash

- Leaving computerized diet sheets on resident trays and dumping them into the general trash after meals

- Posting the documentation form for meal intake on a clipboard on the wall for all to see

- Leaving the meal-intake documentation form unattended in the dining room after meals even though the resident names are covered by a piece of construction paper

- Disclosing identifiable information such as name, address, contact information, medications, medical condition, room number, vitals, etc. (disclosure may be deliberate or inadvertent, such as leaving the computer monitor facing a public area)

- Placing complete names on resident chart covers and leaving the charts in an area in which the public can read resident names

- Taking photos in which residents inadvertently appear in the background

Penalties for violations of the HIPAA rules can be very substantial. The amount and type of penalty are determined by the situation, the safeguards and controls the covered facility has implemented, and the demonstrated and documented compliance efforts made by the facility. Civil monetary penalties (CMP) are enforced by the Department of Health and Human Services.

The U.S. Department of Justice enforces criminal penalties. The fines range from no more than $100 per person for failure to comply with a single regulation up to $25,000 per calendar year per person for recurrent or multiple violations. The penalties increase if violations of multiple regulations or by multiple individuals are identified. Criminal penalties may apply for wrongful disclosure of protected health information.

How to chart

Always follow the documentation policies and procedures established by your employing facility. Most facilities develop policies and procedures based on state law, professional standards of practice, and other requirements, such as those of accrediting organizations. The documentation policies should identify how often documentation should be done, who is responsible for charting in each part of the medical record and what abbreviations, techniques, and procedures are acceptable. If the facility's requirements are less stringent than those of your state nurse practice act, always adhere to the higher standard of the nurse practice act.

- Follow your facility policy for ink color. Most facilities use blue or black ink.

- Follow facility policy for documenting time. Many facilities use military time.

- Chart the exact time treatments, medications, and other procedures were administered, and nursing notes were written. Never document these by using shift times, such as "6-2." Document as soon as possible after care is given.

- Always document the exact time of nursing observations and actions, and physician and family notifications.

- Spell terms correctly, and use proper grammar.

- Illegible entries may adversely affect care and hinder attempts to demonstrate that a reasonable course of treatment was identified and followed. The reader of an illegible entry may infer the care was haphazard or did not meet standards.

- Chart legibly: Sloppy or illegible handwriting can be catastrophic in a lawsuit. If your handwriting is not legible, print.

- Close all entries with your first name or initial, last name, and title. Make sure your signature and title are legible.

- If you initial some entries, such as the medication record, make sure you sign the key with your full signature to match the initials.

- Write the resident's name and other identifying information on each page.

- Avoid skipping lines.

- Chart events in chronological order.

- Be truthful.

- Do not chart in advance or prior to giving care. The only component of the nursing process that may be documented in advance is the plan of care. Document all other observations and activities only after you assess the resident or implement a nursing intervention.

- Document information as close to the time of the event or nursing intervention as possible. If you wait until the end of the shift to document, you may forget important details or eliminate potentially important information because you are pressed for time. If necessary, make notes of important events, and destroy them after documenting in the medical record.

- Use only those abbreviations accepted by your facility. These should be listed in the policy and procedure manual, or other facility manual.

- The Joint Commission and Institute for Safe Medication Practices (ISMP) maintain lists of potentially unsafe abbreviations (see your CD-ROM for a list of these abbreviations). Consider these abbreviations and the rationale for not using them when approving abbreviations for facility documentation.

- Make sure your documentation is in keeping with acceptable nursing practice. Use nursing diagnosis, but avoid making medical diagnoses. Make sure documentation reflects use of the nursing process.

- Document only what you are qualified to do, based on your education, experience, and licensure.

- If a documentation form is more than one page, make sure that all pages are numbered and/or dated so they can be matched up if the chart is dropped, or pages are out of sequence.

What to chart

In the long-term care facility, a complete assessment is not usually done every shift unless the resident is ill or is being monitored. Policies and state laws vary on the frequency of charting, but in stable residents, this is generally weekly or monthly. Daily care, treatments, and medications are usually documented on flow sheets. This is acceptable unless a problem occurs or abnormality develops.

Clinical documentation is the element of resident care that contributes to identification and communication of residents' problems, needs and strengths, that monitors their condition on an ongoing basis, and that records treatment and response to treatment, is a matter of good clinical practice and is an expectation of licensed healthcare professionals.[5] Note that documentation cannot be separated from resident care. It is an element (or part) of comprehensive resident care.

Assessment

Residents who are in the long-term care facility under the Medicare payment program must have a notation on the medical record at least once every 24 hours. However, many facilities require documentation and assessment of the resident's skilled condition and needs each shift. The reason for the policy is usually related to skips in documentation, which is a problem that plagues many long-term care facilities. If a note is required once in 24 hours, and the nurse gets busy, forgets, or otherwise fails to write this note, there is no documentation for the 24-hour period. Thus, most facilities require a note each shift, even if the resident is stable. Remember that the note should reflect the nursing assessment, nursing action, resident response, and evaluation related to the resident's Medicare-covered condition.

If your assessment reveals an abnormality, documentation should describe what nursing action was taken. Simply describing an abnormality is inadequate. In most cases, a notation that simply says, "will continue to monitor" is also inadequate. The nursing process and the plan of care should guide care and documentation. Vague notes referring to ongoing monitoring are not sufficient to describe care or necessary monitoring. Review the steps in the nursing process. Avoid documenting an abnormal observation without documenting the other steps in the nursing process related to this observation. For example, do not document "crackles in lungs" without documenting nursing actions, physician notification, resident response, and follow up evaluation and care. This is a significant issue in many lawsuits.

Record information about allergies and past health history. If the resident has a condition such as arthritis or a pressure ulcer that is potentially painful, document regular pain assessments and nursing interventions to relieve pain. Use an appropriate pain-assessment tool. Avoid random statements, such as, "Smiling. Does not appear to be in pain." For residents with painful or potentially painful conditions, regular assessment is necessary. Failure to assess for, document, or report pain does not mean that residents do not have pain. A quarterly MDS assessment of untreated pain is not adequate.

> The EFG Care Center failed to read the notes and test results authored or written by other healthcare providers and consultant personnel. They failed to recognize the significance of these providers' observations. They apparently overlooked diagnostic reports on the record. They failed to include appropriate management techniques, preventive care, and consultant recommendations on the care plan. They failed to solicit interventions from the consultants for problems experienced by the resident.
>
> These failures deprived the resident of collaborative, interdisciplinary care. (From an actual lawsuit report alleging progressive failures and omissions of care.)

Care given

Remember, you are talking about a person. Review a medical record of a resident with a gastrostomy tube, pressure ulcer, or other chronic condition. Does most of the documentation address the gastrostomy tube or chronic condition to the exclusion of other information about the resident? If so, staff are not documenting holistically. Address the entire person. The condition is always secondary to the person. Use the nursing process.

Nursing facilities are required to document the resident's care and response to care during the course of the stay, and it is expected that this documentation would chronicle, support and be consistent with the findings of each MDS assessment. Always keep in mind that government requirements are not the only or even the major reason for clinical documentation.[6] Charting care that you did not give or assessments you have not done is fraud.

- Make sure your care and documentation are consistent with acceptable professional standards of practice, state laws, facility policies and procedures, and the resident's plan of care.

- Record all nursing care given, including the resident's response to treatment.

- Describe teaching, as well as the resident's response and understanding. List specific instructions you have given.

- Document all safety precautions taken to protect the resident. This may be done on a flow sheet. Be specific. Stating "fall precautions" does not tell the reader what you did. However, listing specific fall precautions on the care plan, then writing precautions per plan of care" may be considered acceptable. However, make sure the plan does not list generic precautions such as "call signal within reach." The plan must be individualized to the resident's needs and updated when necessary.

- Always document the reason for giving a PRN medication and the resident's response.

- When following a physician's order, always leave a "paper trail," e.g., assessment of resident, implementation of valid orders, notification of the physician (and responsible party) and outcome.

EFG Care Center neglected to provide an organizational structure and methodology for the Nursing Services Department to ensure that clinical records were complete, accurate, and contained all necessary information for the care of Donnie Jones. They neglected to develop, maintain, and evaluate a format for documentation that facilitated desired outcomes for Donnie Jones. Documentation is a means of communication with other healthcare providers. EFG Care Center failed to ensure that nurses' notes were informative and descriptive of the resident's condition, care provided, and response to care. They failed to ensure that records were completely and accurately documented. They failed to ensure that nurses assessed intake and output values and compared them with the resident's daily fluid requirements. They failed to ensure that documentation reflected that care was provided within the confines of acceptable professional standards of practice.

Refusals, noncompliance, behavior problems, documenting about the resident and family

- If you document a resident's or family member's comments, place their words in quotation marks and attribute the comment to them. Avoid paraphrasing.

- Document all resident refusals or noncompliance. Cite specific behaviors or statements. The resident has a right to refuse care, but the nurse has a responsibility to explain the consequences of the refusal to the resident in terms he or she can understand. Documentation should reveal adequate teaching.

- Avoid labeling or stereotyping the resident in the medical record.

- Avoid criticizing or expressing animosity toward a resident or family. Describing a resident or family as uncooperative, difficult or manipulative or being sarcastic suggests you do not value or respect the individual. Negative labels, descriptions, and stereotypes may reflect your frustration, but you should make every effort to describe residents and family members factually, in an impartial manner.

- Document the presence of any unauthorized items in the resident's room and action taken.

- Document any actions of the resident or family that contribute to the resident's illness or injury, including refusals of care.

- Refusals of care are often thinly disguised behavior problems. Do adequate teaching to ensure the resident understands the situation completely. Consider trying behavioral approaches. Modify the plan of care to identify and address the behavior. Contact the social worker to see if the resident would benefit from behavior management or mental health services. Don't give up! Document your efforts and results.

- Document tampering with medical equipment, such as oxygen concentrator, IV pump, etc.

- Document the existence and disposition of important personal belongings, large sums of money, and valuables. Add items to the inventory list and ask the resident to sign the list if he or she sends items home. If the family takes items home, remove them from the inventory list and ask the resident or family member to sign the inventory.

- Avoid labeling events and behaviors. Be specific. For example, avoid charting the resident was "uncooperative," or "acting in an unruly manner." Specifically describe the behavior without making judgments. Document conclusions that can be supported with data. You may document observed behavior, such as "refuses bath, shouts and shakes fists."

- Avoid referring to other residents by name. Use words such as "roommate," or refer to the other resident by initial, medical record number, or room number, according to your facility policy.

- If you use an interpreter when instructing a resident, state who the interpreter was and exactly what was discussed. State that you had the resident's consent to communicate the information through the interpreter. Keep explanations simple. Most lay interpreters do not have a medical background and may become confused by technical terminology.

- Document all comments or threats by residents and families, such as, "calling the state," complaining to a professional licensure board, or filing a lawsuit.

Test results, consultations

Document your review of laboratory, radiology, and other reports and note the date, time, and method of physician notification. If you fax an abnormal report to the physician, documentation should reveal that you followed up by telephone in a timely manner. Update the care plan to reflect any monitoring needed for the abnormality. Ask the physician whether follow-up lab is needed.

- The facility must provide or obtain laboratory services to meet the needs of its residents. The facility is responsible for the quality and timeliness of the laboratory services.[7] If laboratory or other test results and reports are not received in a timely manner, document that you notified the appropriate agency, department, or person, and followed up on the situation.

- If the consultant dietitian, pharmacist, or other consultant visits, make sure to read his

- or her notes. Follow up on recommendations. Add changes to the care plan. Contact the physician if orders are necessary. Document his or her response.

EFG Care Center failed to maintain accurate and complete medical records on Donnie Jones. Numerous documents are missing from the record. Minimum Data Sets and care plans are missing from the record. There is no paper trail to verify that some physician orders were followed. Laboratory reports are missing. Facility personnel failed to chronicle physical findings and circumstances leading to Donnie Jones's declines, denying the resident medically necessary care and services.

These examples are not all inclusive; nursing assessment is erratic and largely absent on this record. The medical record is silent relative to a narration of events leading up to the resident's hospitalizations. It is evident from the documentation that nurses were not practicing preventive care or following any type of care plan. Care was inconsistent. Acute conditions were not monitored or acted upon. Care was so fragmented and communication so poor, it appears no one knew what anyone else was doing.

The records were not accessible, information was not communicated and valuable information was not recorded. The record did not give the treating physician sufficient information to make accurate clinical decisions for the resident's care. Examples include, but are not limited to absence of an accurate height measurement, numerous gaps and lack of assessment of intake and output data, numerous care omissions in nursing notes and flow sheets, failure of nursing personnel to address observations made by other providers and documented in the record, and lack of assessment and ongoing monitoring of acute conditions. Weight monitoring is inconsistently documented, erratic, and not done often enough to track the resident's rapid weight loss so it could be promptly addressed and reversed. Weights are contradictory for various documents in the record, such as the MDS, weight record, dietitian's notes, and nursing notes.

There is no evidence that nursing personnel were evaluating and assessing the meaning and significance of the intake numbers they were recording, which is the purpose for monitoring intake and output.

Intake and output

Intake and output (I & O) monitoring does not require a physician's order. However, if the physician orders it, documentation is essential, not optional. Intake and output monitoring, as well as any special approaches or resident preferences are listed on the written care plan. If you list "encourage fluids" as a care plan approach, or if the physician orders increased fluids, you must have a means of evaluating the effectiveness of your approaches. Without a means of evaluation, this approach is meaningless. When documenting I & O, ensure that:

- Fluid intake is planned so that approximately 65%–75% of the total daily intake is delivered at meals, and 25%–35% delivered during nonmeal times, such as medication passes and planned nourishment or snack times. Fluid with medication administration may be standardized to a prescribed amount; e.g., 180 mL (6oz.) per administration pass.

- All fluid the resident consumes during each shift is recorded in metric measurements (cc or mL) on an intake and output flow sheet or worksheet. This includes fluids consumed on the nursing unit, fluids consumed with medications, fluids consumed during meals, and fluids consumed during activities.

- All fluid excreted is also recorded in metric measurements. For the most part, this is urinary elimination. However, emesis, wound drainage, and liquid stools may also be included in output recording.

- The nurse reviews each resident's fluid intake at the end of each shift. If he or she determines that the fluid intake and output are inaccurate or inadequate, he or she will question the accuracy of the recorded information and attempt to reconcile the record. He or she may also instruct the nursing assistant to administer fluids immediately. Low liquid intake may also be reported to the next shift, who will increase fluid intake. Both nurses document the assessment and nursing interventions. Update the plan of care.

Take intake and output monitoring seriously. Make sure the flow sheet is complete. The midnight shift nurse or other designated person should cumulate and assess the 24-hour fluid intake each day. Compare these values with the dietitian's calculations of the resident's minimum fluid requirements. If the resident consumes less than his or her minimum requirements, act on the information! Modify the plan of care to ensure sufficient intake.

Skin condition

Pressure ulcers and skin breakdown are a leading cause of lawsuits against long-term care facilities and their personnel.

- Document the skin risk assessment on admission, quarterly, and according to facility policy. If the resident is at risk, begin a preventive care plan. If the resident experiences new breakdown, repeat the skin assessment promptly.

- If the resident's skin is fragile and at risk for bruises and/or skin tears, implement a protective care plan to prevent injury.

- The standards for monitoring and documenting skin condition include:

  - To prevent pressure ulcers, individuals at risk should be identified so that risk factors can be reduced through intervention. The condition of an individual admitted to a healthcare facility is not static; consequently, pressure ulcer risk requires routine reexamination. Accurate and complete documentation of all risk assessments ensures continuity of care and may be used as a foundation for the skin care plan.[8]

  - All individuals at risk should have a systematic skin inspection at least once a day, paying particular attention to the bony prominences. Results of skin inspection should be documented.[9]

  - Assess the pressure ulcer initially for location, stage, size (length, width, depth), sinus tracts, undermining, tunneling, exudate, necrotic tissue, and the presence or absence of granulation tissue and epithelialization.

  - Reassess pressure ulcers frequently. If the condition of the resident or wound deteriorates, reevaluate the treatment plan as soon as any evidence of deterioration is noted.[10]

  - To achieve successful wound healing, the nurse must carefully follow every step in wound management, including critical assessment, planning, implementation, evaluation, and documentation.[11]

- Facilities should assess and document high-risk residents' skin conditions at least weekly, or more often if breakdown occurs.

- For residents with pressure ulcers or other open skin areas, weekly documentation should reflect at least:

  - Diameter and depth of area, in metric measurements

  - Stage

  - Color

  - Odor (presence or absence of)

  - Drainage (presence or absence of, characteristics, appearance)

- Necrosis (presence or absence of)

- Appearance of the surrounding skin (periphery)

Consistency and objectivity

Documentation must be consistent with the care plan.

- Avoid documenting information that contradicts the approaches listed on the plan.

- Charting should be descriptive. Provide accurate descriptions of information you can see, hear, touch, and smell. Avoid generalizations and vague expressions. Avoid documenting feelings, opinions, or judgments about the resident or his or her family.

- Always document objectively. Avoid terms such as "normal," or "good," "resident had a good night," or "appears" or "seems" which are subjective and can be interpreted many different ways. If you document information such as, "wound healing," or "condition improved," be sure to state facts to support your observation. Give exact measurements and state the observations supporting the opinion.

- Ensure that information about the resident's level of function on the nurses notes' and weekly/monthly summary does not conflict with information in the Minimum Data Set, or other areas of the record. If documentation reflects a change in level of function, clearly state this in the notes. Consider updating the MDS and care plan.

- If a resident is receiving physical, occupational, or speech therapy, make sure that your documentation is consistent. Read what the therapist has written before writing your notes. Conflicting documentation between nursing and therapy is a significant legal and financial issue. It commonly occurs because nurses do not read therapy notes and are not aware of mobility goals. For example, if the therapist notes the resident can safely ambulate in her room with a walker, nursing documentation should not state the resident is routinely restrained in a chair "for safety and to prevent falls." In this case, restraining the resident is effectively reversing the skilled care therapy is providing. If you have concerns about resident safety, meet with the therapist and find a middle ground.

- If a resident is on fall precautions, hip precautions, anticoagulant precautions, or some other type of monitoring, all personnel should be doing the same thing. The facility should have policies and procedures addressing the actions to take. The care plan should state individualized approaches to use for the resident. For example, each nurse notes the resident is on "hip precautions." Without a specific policy or care plan, the reader does not know what precautions were used to protect the resident. This may become an issue if the resident's prosthesis dislocates and he or she is hospitalized and promptly dies of a pulmonary embolus.

- Documentation in one part of the medical record should be consistent and not contradict information in other parts. For example, a resident's weight is recorded as 123 pounds on the October 1 MDS. The October 3 dietitian note documents the resident's weight as 92 pounds. The nursing summary of October 5 states the resident weighs 114 pounds. The flow sheet of October 7 states the resident weighs 98 pounds. The magnitude of the inconsistencies makes it clear that no one knows the resident's true weight. In extreme cases, facilities may be charged with Medicare or Medicaid fraud because they were paid for care that was not provided. At the very least, the personnel in this facility do not appear credible, based on the erratic, inconsistent, contradictory documentation, and there is no clear benefit to the resident.

- When charting, emphasize quality of content, not quantity of words.

Cosigning and documenting for others

Follow these guidelines when cosigning and documenting for others:

- As a rule, do not document for someone else.

- Avoid adding information to someone else's notes.

- Do not change or correct someone else's charting. If you discover that a coworker has made an error, do not correct it. Inform that person about the error. Correcting someone else's documentation is a legal issue that can cause serious problems if the medical record goes to court.

- Avoid cosigning documentation if you cannot attest to the accuracy of the information.

Documentation must reflect who performed the action. If it is absolutely necessary to document care given by another person, document factual information. For example, the nurse from the previous shift calls and states she gave a resident acetaminophen for arthritic pain several minutes before her shift ended and forgot to document it. In this case, making a narrative note explaining the details of the nurse's notification is appropriate. Assess and document the resident's current level of pain. Initial the medication record with "your initials for (the other nurse's initials)." When the nurse arrives for her next shift, she should cosign this documentation.

You have asked that I review the medical records of Donnie Jones, which your office provided. These records were made and maintained by the EFG Care Center. No other medical records were received or reviewed in connection with the care of this resident. The EFG Care Center records are incomplete. They begin on December 29, 2004. The nursing notes end on March 3, 2005. Notes for March 4, 2005 are missing. The progress notes and physician orders end on March 4, 2005, which appears to be the actual date of discharge from the facility. The dates of service are missing from the various consultation reports on the record. The resident sustained a fall and serious hip fracture in the facility on January 12, 2005. All nursing notes for this day have been removed from the record. When a medical record is altered, sanitized or tampered with, it calls the credibility/integrity and veracity of the entire document into question.

Countersigning someone else's documentation generally means the nurse has verified that all required resident care has been provided. In some facilities, nursing assistants are not permitted to write in the narrative notes. Their care and observations are documented on flow sheets, with additional narrative information entered on nurses' notes by the licensed nurse. Activities of daily living flow sheets are commonly completed by nursing assistants each shift. The forms may be reviewed and countersigned by a nurse. Facility policies should address the meaning of countersigned documentation; i.e., whether by documenting on a flow sheet the licensed nurse is verifying the care was provided, or simply that the nursing assistant had the authority and competence to perform the procedure.[12]

Some facilities require nurses to complete the ADL flow sheets because of problems with documentation errors and skips by nursing assistants. Consult the facility legal counsel about this practice. It is virtually impossible for the nurse to know that each item he or she signs off represents care that was given as documented. This is an example of documenting care that is supposed to be given without knowing it was actually given. It may cause the reader to question the veracity, integrity, and credibility of the nurses' documentation. Document care only if you gave it personally, or directly and personally observed an unlicensed worker providing the care.

Master signature legends for flow sheets

Unless prohibited by state law, facilities are permitted to maintain master signature legends as a key to the initials on flow sheets. This eliminates the need for personnel to sign a signature key for each flow sheet every month. However, in facilities with heavy turnover, tracking the signatures of employees daily to ensure the master signature legend is accurate may be impossible. The federal requirements state that use of a master signature legend in lieu of the legend on each form for nursing staff signatures of medication, treatment, or flow sheet entries is acceptable under the following circumstances:[13]

- Each nursing employee documenting on medication, treatment, or flow sheets signs his full name, title, and initials on the legend.

- The original master legend is kept in the clinical records office or director of nurses' office.

- A current copy of the legend is filed at each nurses' station.

- When a nursing employee leaves employment with the facility, his name is deleted from the list by lining through it and writing the current date by the name.

- The facility updates the master legend as needed for newly hired and terminated employees.

- The master signature legend must be retained permanently as a reference to entries made in clinical records.

If your facility maintains a master signature legend, consult your legal counsel to determine whether you must furnish a copy of the legends for the relevant time frame when a resident requests a copy of his or her medical record. If lawsuit is filed, the plaintiff attorney will most probably subpoena these records if you have not previously furnished them. He or she may also subsequently subpoena time cards, assignment sheets, schedules, personnel files, and other employee data.

The medical-legal reviewer will compare initials on the signature legends with the flow sheets. If he or she questions the veracity of the record or suspects falsification of the flow sheets or other information, the reviewer may compare the initials, names, handwriting, signatures, or other data with schedules, assignment sheets, time cards, and payroll data to confirm whether certain individuals were employed and on duty during the days in question.

Staffing problems, problems with other workers:

- Keep comments about other staff members or allegations of inadequate care out of the record.

- Avoid documenting information about staffing shortages, criticisms of the employer, problems, or conflicts in the resident's medical record, such as "Treatment not done due to lack of staff."

- Avoid criticizing other healthcare workers in the record.

- Avoid stating you have "informed" a supervisor, physician, or other healthcare provider of an event if you have barely mentioned it, or mentioned it briefly in passing.

- Transfers and discharges.

- When a resident leaves your care, document the time, the condition of the resident upon leaving, and any other information necessary to reflect the situation accurately. For example, if the resident is at risk for skin breakdown, document the complete condition of the skin.

- When transferring a resident, state the date and time, resident condition, who accompanied the resident, who provided the transfer, where and to whom the resident is transferred, and manner of transfer (wheelchair, stretcher, ambulance, and so forth). Document the disposition of the resident's personal possessions and medications. List instructions given to the resident, and teaching in anticipation of discharge.

Readmissions

If a resident is discharged for 30 days or fewer and readmitted to the same facility, the medical record must be updated upon readmission. To update the clinical record, staff must:

- Obtain current, signed physicians' orders.

- Completely assess the resident's condition using the facility admission assessment form and/or write a descriptive nursing note, giving a complete assessment of the resident's condition.

- Note changes in diagnoses, if any.

- Obtain signed copies of the hospital or transferring facility history and physical and discharge summary, if applicable. A signed transfer form containing this information is acceptable, but may not be as complete as the other documents.

- Complete a new RAI and update the comprehensive care plan if evaluation of the resident reveals a significant change that appears to be permanent. If no significant change has occurred, then update only the comprehensive care plan.

- If the resident has been discharged from the facility for more than 30 days, a new clinical record must be initiated.

Late entries, addendums, clarifications

Adhere to the following advice when documenting late entries, addendums, and clarifications:

- Late entries are acceptable if the delay is justified by the circumstances. The documentation should never appear to be self-serving.

- If you forget to document, follow your facility policy for making a late entry. Specify the exact date and time the entry was recorded, as well as the exact date and time the event occurred.

- Clearly mark your documentation as a "Late entry for (date, time)."

Avoid making late entries or rewriting new pages of the record to make the details sound more favorable. This is usually a transparent attempt to cover up negative outcomes. You may add late entry information if it pertains to information and missing details. However, making details sound favorable in a late entry gives the reader the impression that you are hiding something. An attorney or jury may assume that the information was added for damage control purposes.

A clarification note is a late entry that is written to prevent incorrect interpretation of information that has been previously documented. For example, after reading an entry, you can see how it could be easily misinterpreted. Write the clarification note as soon after the original entry as possible. To make a clarification entry, note the current date and time. Write "clarification." State the reason for the clarification and refer to the entry being clarified. Identify any additional documents or sources of information that support the clarification.

If you must add something to a previously written entry, go to the next available line and write, "Addendum to note of (date and time of prior note)." An addendum is a late entry that provides new or additional information related to a previous entry. The addendum refers to the previous note and provides additional information to address a specific situation or incident. Refer to information supporting the addendum, if any. Do not use this type of note if you forget to chart something. (Use a late entry for forgotten information.) To make an addendum, note the current date and time. Write "addendum" and state the reason, referring to the previous documentation. Complete the addendum entry as soon as possible.

Errors, omissions, and corrections

If you make an error, do not erase it, use correction fluid, or otherwise obliterate it. Avoid writing over the entry to correct it. The original entry must be visible. Draw a single, thin line through the entry, and write "error." Sign your name, and initial and date the change. State the reason for the error, such as "wrong chart" in the margin or above the note. Then write the correct information. If someone else has made a subsequent entry, skip down to the next available line and write the correction as a late entry, referring to the previous incorrect entry.

Check the medication record, treatment record, and flow sheets at the end of your shift to make sure you have documented all information for which you were responsible.

Be aware that there are many pitfalls with checklist and flow-sheet charting. Initial care only if you personally completed it. Don't follow the previous nurse's checkmarks and don't chart care unless you know it was actually done. Be aware that blank spaces in flow sheets raise doubts about whether or not something was done. If a resident is in the hospital or out of the facility, remove the sheet from the notebook or turn it over or upside down until the resident returns.

Do not chart care because it is supposed to be done. Chart only if care was actually given. For example, avoid blanket statements, such as "turned q two hours," "peri care after each incontinence," "toileted q2h," "call light within reach," etc. unless you personally know that this was done as documented throughout the shift. Many nurses document this information because it is "supposed to be done." The medical record is a true, complete, and accurate record of care given. Thus, care that is "supposed to be done" does not belong in the record, and may undermine the nurses' credibility. In some facilities, nurses complete activities of daily living flow sheets. This, too, is a questionable practice because in most cases, the nurse does not give this care and does conclusively know what care has been provided. In a courtroom, you can expect this type of documentation to be scrutinized and questioned by the plaintiff attorney.

If you make an omission or mistake, it must be documented. Document only the facts, which will speak for themselves. Avoid making statements such as, "I made a mistake," or "the nursing assistant made an error." Other words to avoid are "accidentally," "somehow," or "inadvertently."

Practice defensive documentation, but avoid lying or selectively omitting potentially damaging information.

Document omitted medications and treatments. Circle them on the flow sheet to indicate they were not given. State the reason in a narrative note or on the back of the flow sheet.

Occasionally, documentation is lost. If you must recreate an entry because of missing or lost information, clearly mark the entry as a replacement for lost information. If you cannot recall the event or care, state that information for the specific time frame has been lost.

When documentation spans two pages (continues from one page to the next), always sign your name and title at the bottom of the first page. Note that the entry will "continue on the next page." Begin the new page by noting the date and time from the previous page. Note that the entry is "continued from previous page." Write the resident's identifying information in the appropriate space on the new form.

Falsification

Be truthful in your documentation. Although you may practice defensive documentation do not omit or alter relevant details of any event.

Tampering with, altering, or falsifying the medical record in any manner is fraud. Any individual tampering with a medical record is subject to criminal, civil, and licensure action. Fraud has a longer statute of limitations than medical malpractice in some states. The nursing licensure board is not bound to the statute of limitations when investigating and punishing nurses for fraudulent documentation. Also:

- Never record care you have not given. Avoid making up or overstating information. Avoid documentation that is obviously self-serving.

- Do not alter or destroy the medical record.

- Do not remove and rewrite pages of the medical record. On rare occasions, liquid or another substance may be spilled on a medical record, or a page may be damaged so it is illegible. If this is the case, retain the original page. Make the reason for recopying clear. Mark it as damaged and on what date. Recopy the page exactly like the original. Place both pages in the chart, or note where the damaged original is located. This prevents concern that a page was recopied to conceal or add information.

- You may feel pressured to fill in gaps in flow sheet charting. This is a dangerous practice because you may not remember what occurred several weeks after the fact. Completing flow sheets during your shift is always best. If gaps in flow sheets are a problem in your facility, assign someone to audit them each shift. Going back and completing or "filling holes" in the medication, treatment, or ADL flow sheets is considered willful falsification and is illegal. Facility policies should address how to correct omissions on flow sheets, but only if the person making the correction has complete and total recall of the care given. Some states have time frames in which omissions may be completed. Usually, you cannot go back and correct a flow sheet. Writing a late entry narrative note describing the care given is probably the best approach.

- Charting medication administration, treatments, or other care in advance is falsification of records.

- Writing your initials on a medication record indicates the medication has been given, not just removed from the drawer. (The same principle applies for all other flow sheet charting.)

- If you place your initials on the record before giving the medication, you are increasing your risk of legal exposure. (The same principle applies for all other flow sheet charting.)

- Evidence of tampering with a chart not only is illegal, it can cause the entire medical record to be inadmissible as evidence in court.[14]

Medical record accuracy

Medical records and documentation are not only part of the resident's care, they are the validation of that care. Without accurate and complete documentation, no one can really determine what has been done or what should be a future clinical approach to resident care.[15] If you are involved in a lawsuit or questioned by an attorney, avoid using the excuse that documentation is a bureaucratic requirement that adds nothing to the resident's care or well-being. The opposing attorney is bound to have an expert witness who will persuasively explain why properly maintained medical records are important and essential to the residents' welfare.

Make sure that your documentation is accurate. Errors, omissions, and questionable or inaccurate entries diminish your credibility. This is an issue if the nursing care is questioned or negligence is alleged, affecting both the reliability of your chart and the strength of your case if you end up in court. Covering up minor errors that were not negligent damages your credibility. An accurate and concise record shows you are conscientious. It implies that you have given quality care. Errors suggest you are careless. If you are careless with your documentation, the reader may assume you are careless with the care you give.

Medical record retention

The facility is required by law to safeguard clinical records against loss, destruction, or unauthorized use. The facility must keep confidential all information in the resident's records, regardless of the form or storage method of the records, unless release is required by:

- Law

- Transfer to another healthcare institution

- Third-party payment contract

- The resident

Formal facility medical record retention policies are determined by state law. If your state law does not specify a period of time for which to retain records, the facility must keep them for five years after the date of the resident's discharge. If the resident is a minor, retain records for at least three years after the resident's 21st birthday, or the legal age according to state law.

Thinning charts

Nursing personnel are often required to "thin" the active medical records to fit in the charts. Forms that have been removed are sent to the medical records department, where they are maintained in each resident's permanent file. If a record is requested by a resident or law firm, check the thinning pile to make sure the resident's thinned records have all been filed in the resident's permanent file. Certain forms must remain on the open chart permanently, whereas others may be removed and filed after a period of time. Most facilities retain three to six months of departmental notes on the open record. Facilities are strongly encouraged to provide written guidelines for staff for thinning their open charts. The following items must remain in the active clinical record (open chart):

- Current history and physical

- Current physicians' orders

- Current physician progress notes

- All RAIs and Quarterly Reviews for the previous 15-month period

- Current care plan

- Most recent hospital discharge summary and/or transfer form

- Current nursing and therapy notes

- Current medication and treatment records

- Current lab and x-ray reports

- The admission record

- The current permanency plan

The facility must maintain a permanent, master index of all residents admitted to and discharged from the facility. This index must contain at least the following information:

- Name of resident (first, middle, and last)

- Date of birth

- Date of admission

- Date of discharge

- Social security, Medicare, or Medicaid number

Destruction of records

When resident records are destroyed after the retention period is complete, the facility should shred or incinerate the records in a manner that protects resident confidentiality. At the time of record destruction, maintain a log to document the following for each record destroyed:

- Resident name

- Date of birth

- Medical record number

- Social security number, Medicare/Medicaid number. A master index can be found on your CD-ROM.

- Date and signature of person disposing of the record

- Method of record disposal

Facility closure

In the event the facility closes, changes ownership, or changes administrative authority, the new management must maintain documented proof of the medical information required for all residents. This documentation may be in the form of copies of the resident's clinical record or the original clinical record. In a change of ownership, the two parties will agree and designate in writing who will be responsible for the retention and protection of the inactive and closed clinical records.

Communication books, shift reports, anecdotal records

Communication books and shift reports are used to alert the healthcare team to critical information. These tools should note where the relevant information is documented. Relevant health information documented in these tools must also be documented in the health record. Nurses may use personal or anecdotal notes to record personal reflections and resident information. This information must also be documented in the residents' charts. Personal and anecdotal notes can be requested during legal proceedings.

- Use communication books and shift reports only for information that must be passed on to other members of the healthcare team.

- Pertinent information from communication books and shift reports must also be included in the residents' records.

- Maintain resident confidentiality when storing or disposing of communication books, shift reports, anecdotal records, such as by destroying or shredding the documents.

- Follow facility policies for retaining and storing communication books, shift reports, schedules, assignment sheets, and other internal documents in a secure area for a specified period of time.

Evaluating your documentation

Since nurses are responsible for assigning and delegating to nursing assistants, the nurse is responsible for monitoring nursing assistant documentation to ensure it is accurate and complete. All facilities should set a goal for random chart audits quarterly. This shows staff that management is concerned with documentation substance, accuracy, and completion. When trying to determine whether your charting meets acceptable professional standards, ask yourself:

- Are your medical records as complete as they should be to fully document what you did and why, including the resident's response?

- Does your documentation reveal each element of the nursing process?

- Does your documentation reveal that the residents' risks and needs were identified, and care was given to meet these needs?

- Does your documentation reveal you followed the care plan?

- Does your documentation contradict information elsewhere on the record, including the MDS?

- Does your documentation reflect care that was actually given (versus care that is supposed to be given)?

- Does your documentation clearly show evidence of evaluations and outcomes (even if outcomes differ from stated goals or include deviations from normal)?

- Would a plaintiff attorney or expert be able to criticize you?

- Would a defense attorney or expert be able to defend you?

- Would Medicare or Medicaid agree that your note justifies the care they paid for?

- Does documentation validate a higher level of care and a higher payment rate?

Example electronic media policy

Employees have access to various forms of electronic media and services (computers, e-mail, telephones, voicemail, fax machines, external electronic bulletin boards, wire services, online services, and the Internet (hereinafter called "media").

The facility encourages the use of electronic media. However, media provided by the facility are facility property and the purpose of the devices is to transact facility business.

The following procedures apply to all media that are:

- Accessed on or from facility premises

- Accessed using facility computer equipment or via facility-paid access methods

- Individually identifiable, including communications that make reference to the facility in any manner; and/or

- Used in a manner that identifies the employee with the facility

Media may not be used for transmitting, retrieving, or storing any communications that are of a discriminatory or harassing nature; derogatory to any individual or group; obscene; of a defamatory or threatening nature; for "chain letters"; for personal use; illegal or against facility policy; or contrary to the facility's interest.

Electronic information created and/or communicated by an employee using media will not generally be monitored by the facility. However, the facility routinely monitors usage patterns for both voice and data communications (e.g., number called or site accessed; call length; times of day called) for cost analysis/allocation and the management of the Internet server. The facility also reserves the right, in its discretion, to review any employee's electronic files and messages and usage to the extent necessary to ensure that media are being used in compliance with the law and with facility policy. Therefore, employees should not assume electronic communications are private and confidential.

Employees must respect other people's electronic communications. Employees may not attempt to read or "hack" into other systems or logins; "crack" passwords; breach computer or network security measures; or monitor electronic filings or communications of other employees or third parties except by explicit direction of facility management.

Every employee who uses any security measures on a facility-supplied computer must provide the facility with a sealed envelope containing a hard copy record of all passwords and encryption keys (if any) for facility use if required.

No e-mail or other electronic communications may be sent that attempt to conceal the identity of the sender or represent the sender as someone else or someone from another facility.

Media may not be used in a manner that is likely to cause network congestion or significantly hamper the ability of other people to access and use the system.

Employees may not copy, retrieve, modify, or forward copyrighted materials except as permitted by the copyright owner or except for a single copy for reference use only.

Any information or messages sent by an employee via an electronic network are statements identifiable and attributable to the facility. All communications sent by employees via a network must comply with facility policy, and may not disclose any confidential or proprietary facility information.

Network services and World Wide Web sites monitor access and usage and can identify at least which facility and often which specific individual is accessing their services. Accessing a particular bulletin board or Web site leaves facility-identifiable electronic "tracks" even if the employee merely reviews or downloads the material and does not post any message.

Any employee violating this policy will be subject to corrective action and/or risk losing the privilege of using media for him/herself and possibly other employees.

Employees are responsible for keeping virus protection up to date by downloading weekly computer updates. Employees must virus-scan all file attachments before opening them.

Employees must use discretion in opening files. Avoid indiscriminate opening of files attached to email. In general, do not open files with the suffix ".exe." Notify the information technology manager if a file with this suffix is received. You must avoid all files if you are not familiar with the sender or are not expecting the file. Employees may be held responsible for the cost of repairs for damage to computers caused by opening files infected with viruses. Employees will be subject to disciplinary action if data is lost as a result of viral infection of the computer.

Example policy for personal communication

It is the policy of this facility to prohibit the use by staff and students of non-work-related personal communication devices, including but not limited to cell phones, pagers, text messaging units, PDAs, and TPCs. Safety and care of the residents is paramount. The cessation of work, even briefly, to make or answer telephone calls or to check an electronic pager or other wireless communication device is not consistent with this goal. In nonclinical departments, use of personal communication devices may represent a safety hazard and interferes with your work. Honesty demands that time paid by the employer will be used profitably. If the work assigned is insufficient to occupy the time, report to the nurse in charge or other supervisor for additional duties. Please plan to make and return all personal communications and phone calls during breaks only.

In addition to being a distraction, the use of camera phones present opportunities for serious violations of residents' rights to confidentiality, dignity, and privacy. Taking still photographs or making videotapes of residents with camera phones or other personal electronic equipment is strictly prohibited.

Generally speaking, do not bring personal communication devices to the work area. These may be accidentally lost, damaged, or broken when on duty. Some radio frequency devices will interfere with medical equipment and may jeopardize resident health and safety, as well as facility operations. Employees must accept responsibility for informing family and friends and asking them to comply with this policy. Disruptions of work or resident care by personal communication devices is grounds for discipline or termination. The facility is not responsible for damage to or loss of personal communication devices.

We understand that emergencies may occur, and these will be accommodated, if possible. If a situation arises in which communication is critical, speak with your supervisor. He or she has the discretion to approve a one-time, acceptable compromise to this policy. (Situations such as "the babysitter may need to get ahold of me" are generally not considered emergencies, and may be handled by calling the facility in the usual manner.) In extraordinary circumstances, the supervisor may agree to the temporary use of an electronic pager or cellular phone set for silent alert that is imperceptible to others. In these situations, the staff member will not interrupt resident care to respond to calls, but rather will respond after resident comfort and safety are assured.

Contents of the medical record

Information in the medical record falls into six general categories:

- Medical findings, and/or information about the resident's condition

- Assessments and identification of risk factors and problems requiring care

- The care plan and documentation of care treatment given to meet the residents' basic needs and address the problems

- Evidence that care follows applicable standards and the care/treatment plan

- Goals of care and evaluation of outcomes achieved/resident response to care

- Effectiveness of the care/treatment plan and modification of the plan when needed

The information is located in many different places in the medical record. Most long-term care facilities use a system called source oriented medical records (SOMR). The SOMR is divided into categories, such as physician orders and progress notes, nurses' notes, vital signs and weights, medications, treatments, laboratory and other diagnostic data, dietary, therapy, social services, and activities. Each category or discipline has a separate divider in the chart in which their records are stored. The sequence of the record is determined by facility or corporate policy and varies from one facility to the next. Most file forms are backwards chronological order, with most recent records on top.

Some facilities use the problem-oriented medical record (POMR). This type of record is divided into general categories, such as history, encounters, orders, progress notes, and test results. In some facilities, the record is subdivided into anatomic categories. All disciplines chart in each category, as appropriate. Facilities that use this system believe it improves communication and makes finding information easier. The structure of the POMR readily translates to electronic documentation, and has been used efficiently in many electronic medical record environments, including those that are highly specialized.

Discharge planning

Nursing facilities are required to develop a post-discharge plan of care when the resident will be transferred to another facility, or to his or her own home. This requirement is the source of a great deal of confusion, and many deficiencies on surveys. The requirement does not apply if the resident is transferred to the acute care hospital in an emergency and does not return to the facility.

Discharge planning begins on facility admission and continues throughout the resident's stay in the facility. If the resident subsequently transfers to another facility or to his or her own home, the facility should:

- Prepare a post-discharge plan of care.

- Teach the resident and/or responsible party about the care plan, as applicable. Give them a copy of the plan of care. Also provide written instructions, if needed, and essential phone numbers to call for problems or questions.

- Send a copy of the most recent MDS and other relevant documents if the resident is being transferred to another long-term care facility.

The standard:
F283 (e) Discharge Summary: When the facility anticipates discharge a resident must have a discharge summary that includes—

F283 (1) A recapitulation of the resident's stay;

(2) A final summary of the resident's status to include items in paragraph (b)(2)* of this section, at the time of discharge that is available for release to authorized persons and agencies, with the consent of the resident or legal representatives; and

F284 (3) A post-discharge plan of care that is developed with the participation of the resident and his or her family, which will assist the resident to adjust to his or her new living environment.

The interpretive guidelines, which are guidance for surveyors in determining whether a deficiency exists, state at §483.20(e)

- A post-discharge plan of care for an anticipated discharge applies to a resident whom the facility discharges to a private residence, to another nursing facility or skilled nursing facility, or to another type of residential facility such as a board-and-care home or an intermediate care facility for mentally retarded individuals. Resident protection concerning transfer and discharge are found at 42 CFR 483.12. A "post-discharge plan of care" means the discharge planning process that includes assessing continuing care needs and developing a plan designed to ensure the individual's needs will be met after discharge from the facility into the community.

- "Anticipates" means the discharge was not an emergency discharge (e.g. hospitalization for an acute condition) or due to the resident's death.

- "Adjust to his or her new living environment" means the post-discharge plan, as appropriate, should describe the resident's and family's preferences for care, how the resident and family will contact these services, and how care should be coordinated if continuing treatment involves multiple caregivers. It should identify specific resident needs after discharge such as personal care, sterile dressings, and physical therapy, as well as describe resident/caregiver education needs to prepare the resident for discharge.

- In plain language, surveyors often interpret this to mean that a discharge care plan will be developed and reviewed with the resident and/or responsible party.

- A copy of the plan is sent to the receiving facility or agency, or home with the family caregiver. For legal purposes, the facility should retain a copy of the discharge care plan, transfer form, and all related documents on the resident's closed medical record.

- The items referred to include information about the resident's medical condition and previous medical history, physical and mental status, sensory and physical impairments, nutritional status and requirements, special treatments or procedures, mental or psychosocial status, dental condition, activities, cognitive status, rehabilitation potential, discharge potential, and drug therapy.

- Another caveat that may be overlooked is "Any time a resident is admitted to a new facility (regardless of whether or not it is a transfer within the same chain), a new comprehensive assessment must be done within 14 days. When transferring a resident, the transferring facility must give the new facility necessary medical records, including appropriate MDS assessments, to support the continuity of resident care."[16]

Records from other facilities

If the resident transferred from your facility to a hospital or another long-term care facility, you can expect the plaintiff attorney to request their records as well. The resident's condition upon arrival is very important to the initial medical-legal record review.

The electronic medical record

Facilities that use electronic documentation are required to have a backup system from which records can be reconstructed in the event the computer goes down. They are also required to have a secure system so unauthorized individuals cannot access the resident information. Each person using the computer must have an individual electronic identifier. This is usually done by maintaining a user name and password.

When documenting electronically, a few additional precautions are in order:

- Don't be afraid of computerized charting.

- Keep in mind that audit trails track the computer, user, date, time, and exactly which medical records are accessed based on the user identification. In many programs, the computer's internal clock automatically documents the date and time of the entry.

- When documenting on a specific resident, double check to make sure you have entered the correct identification code.

- Some computers display a greeting when you log on. The greeting will note the last date and time you logged onto the computer. Always read this message. If the greeting shows you logged on for a day when you were not on duty, report this security breach immediately.

- Use only your own identification and password. Never use someone else's.

- Select a password that is not easily deciphered. Avoid dates such as your birth date or anniversary. A combination of letters and numbers is very effective, such as "83PF211UTK."

- Do not give your identification code or password to others. Do not write it down and leave it under the mouse pad, keyboard, or in an electronic file. Change your password periodically. Change the password immediately if you suspect it has been compromised. Remember it!

- Do not let someone look over your shoulder when you are logging on or accessing resident data.

- Protect confidential information displayed on monitors (e.g., location of monitor, use of screen saver, privacy screens).

- Access only information you are authorized to obtain, and is necessary for you to know.

- Document only in areas you are authorized to use.

- Protect resident confidentiality if information is also reproduced in hard copy. Do not print information unnecessarily. Destroy printed copies that are not part of the permanent record.

- Never delete information from the computerized record.

- Many computer programs place expert reminders or error codes on the screen. Read and follow the directions given.

- The procedure for late entry and addendum documentation will be different than it is in a narrative system. Know and follow your facility policies for this type of charting.

- To correct an error in an electronic medical record, you will follow the same basic principles as a manual system. The computer will be able to track corrections or changes after documentation has been authenticated. Enter the current date and time, identify yourself, and state the reason for the change. If a hard copy has been generated, it must also be corrected.

- The facility must maintain a hard copy of each resident's MDS, even if the clinical record system is entirely electronic. The MDS must be signed by the RN and each individual who has completed a portion of the assessment.

- Always log off when you have finished using the computer.

- Always wash your hands immediately after using the computer. Many people use it, so the keyboard is a potential source of cross contamination.

- Some facilities cover the keyboard with a plastic cover. Users type through the plastic. If this is the case, the cover should be routinely disinfected. (However, prompt hand-washing is still necessary after you have used the computer.)

- When cleaning the computer and accessories, avoid products containing alcohol. Use only products that are recommended for the surface being cleaned.

- The electronic record must note whether manual records are also being used. Likewise, if a manual record is used during an electronic system failure, the records must cross reference each other.

- When data from a manual record is entered into a computerized record, the entry should identify who documented and who provided the care.

- Electronic documentation must be signed by the person providing care. Electronic signatures are valid provided that they are accessible only to the person identified by that signature.

- Protect resident data transmitted electronically, such as by using an e-mail encryption service.

- Stay current. Attend continuing education programs to learn how to maximize the use of computerized charting and information systems.

Electronic data transmission

Electronic data transmission via fax (facsimile) or e-mail (electronic mail) is acceptable for sending and receiving healthcare information, documents, laboratory reports, physician notifications, and physicians' orders. Most facilities routinely transmit RAI information to a state regulatory office over the internet.

If the nature of an electronic communication is urgent, you may want to notify the receiving party by phone to expect the arrival of an urgent fax transmission. With a nonurgent fax, it is also a good idea to call the intended recipient to notify him or her to expect a facsimile. You may also want to consider asking the recipient to send a return fax to verify the information was received.

When sending information by electronic means, long-term care facilities should:

- Implement safeguards to assure that faxed documents are directed to the correct location to protect confidential health information.

- Sign all faxed documents before transmission.

- Set your fax machine to print a verification report for each fax transmission; maintain a file or log of these reports.

- Check to make sure you have the correct fax number before dialing. Read the number on the fax machine display after you have entered it. Recheck the number again before pressing the send button.

- If you believe the fax went to the wrong number, contact the recipient and apologize for the inconvenience, or send another fax asking the recipient to destroy the material.

- Never transmit insecure, identifiable resident information.

- Use the subject line of the email or cover sheet for the fax to warn the receiver that the transmission contains confidential data. On the fax cover sheet, clearly note in large, bold letters that the accompanying material is confidential.

- Place a disclaimer in the body of the e-mail or in large letters at the bottom of the fax cover sheet.

Handheld computers and HIPAA compliance

Personal digital assistants (PDAs) and Tablet PCs (TPCs) are handheld computers that have become quite popular in recent years. Some staff members have purchased the units for personal use, but also use them to record data while at work. In addition to using the computer as an information resource at work, most individuals use them as a source of personal information, such as their appointments, important addresses, and list of phone numbers. Most also have a calculator function. Computers are very beneficial, and the portability of handheld models has made them a popular alternative.

In some facilities, handheld computers are used to transmit data using wireless internet technology. Thus, the facility may transmit sensitive information such as ADL flow sheet data, neuro checks, intake and output values, pain-scale ratings, nursing notes and vital signs to the mainframe computer. Before handheld computer technology was available, nursing personnel commonly scribbled notes on the backs of their hands, on paper towels, and scraps of paper. If the data were not subsequently lost, they were transferred to resident charts later in the shift. By using the handheld computer, personnel can record important data by typing on the keypad with a stylus, then transmitting it to the main computer. Light pens and touch-screen data entry are also useful tools with some models. The handheld device is not practical for long entries, but as you can see, the unit can hold a wealth of PHI for each resident. It can be plugged into a regular keyboard for typing longer narrative entries.

The handheld computer is portable, and operates by using a rechargeable battery. Hot-syncing is a term that refers to linking the handheld computer to a full-size computer to update the information on both. The PDA is placed in a cradle and a button is pushed to upload data to the mainframe. Placing the unit into the cradle also recharges the battery.

HIPAA affects all healthcare communication, and information technology (IT) contains a wealth of information. Because of this, facilities usually have layers of access to resident medical records. The IT department will have a system for tracking who is accessing any resident's record, and will be able to identify misuse of the system.

When PDAs and TPCs are used in the facility, the following potential problems must be anticipated and addressed:

- Important resident data will be lost if the unit is not regularly charged and maintained. Anticipate battery use in advance and make sure data is transferred to the mainframe before the battery goes dead.

- Since PDAs and TPCs usually have the ability to access the Internet wirelessly, the facility must construct and maintain a firewall that is strong enough to ensure that sensitive resident data are not being broadcast into cyberspace.

- Although PDAs and TPCs have enormous benefit and many potential applications in healthcare facilities, protection of resident confidentiality and maintaining HIPAA compliance may be a drawback. Make sure wireless internet transmissions are protected by a firewall. Policies and procedures must address personal use of the devices outside of the facility. Taking PHI home in the computer and inadvertently allowing family members and others to access it is a serious HIPAA violation. Personal computers used at work must have encryption, passwords, and other safeguards to prevent others (including your own family members) from accessing the resident data.

Requests for medical records

Each facility should have specific policies, procedures, consents, and authorization forms for medical record release upon request of the resident or responsible party. You may wish to write a sentence into your policies, such as notifying the facility administrator or facility legal counsel any time a record has been requested. Do not send the records out until he or she gives approval. However, you have a tight time frame to respond, so do not delay making contact. The resident or his or her legal representative has the right:

- Upon an oral or written request, to access all records pertaining to himself or herself including current clinical records within 24 hours (excluding weekends and holidays)

- After receipt of his or her records for inspection, to purchase at a cost not to exceed the community standard photocopies of the records or any portions of them upon request and two working days advance notice to the facility.

In addition to clinical records, the term "records" includes all records pertaining to the resident, such as trust fund ledgers, admission agreements, and contracts between the resident and the facility. "Purchase" is a charge to the resident for photocopying. If state statute has defined the "community standard" rate, facilities should follow that rate. In the absence of state statute, the "cost not to exceed the community standard" is that rate charged per copy by organizations such as the public library, the Post Office or a commercial copy center, which would be selected by a prudent buyer in addition to the cost of the clerical time needed to photocopy the records.

Additional fees for locating the records or typing forms/envelopes may not be assessed.[17] When determining what to charge, make sure to recover your costs for the materials. A large, high-volume commercial copy center buys products in bulk and often gets a discounted rate. You may find you cannot recover the cost of toner when charging the rate a commercial copy center charges.

Some facilities charge for each page, such as 10 to 50 cents a page. Others charge 75 cents to a dollar a page. Some have package prices, such as:

- A basic retrieval or processing fee not to exceed $30.00 for first 10 pages of records; then,

   a. $1.00 per page for pages 11-60.

   b. $.50 per page for pages 61-400.

c. $.25 per page for any remaining pages.

d. Plus actual cost of mailing or shipping.

e. In addition, a reasonable fee not to exceed $10.00 is charged for execution of an affidavit or certification of records.

f. Microform or electronic medium copy processing fee can be up to $45.00.

g. You may also charge for the costs of mailing if it is being mailed to another location.

Although most facilities prefer a signed release to produce medical records, the federal rules state that an oral request may be sufficient to produce the current record for review. You may still request a written release, but do not withhold records if the individual requesting the records does not sign it. Most facilities use a records release form such as, "Authorization for Release of Medical Information."

The release must be dated and signed before records are provided. Make sure the form is time-limited, with an expiration date for medical record release, such as 30 days, 60 days, or 90 days. If another copy is requested after the specified time period, a new authorization should be signed and dated by the appropriate party. The written consent must specify the:

- Information or specific medical records covered by the release

- Reasons or purposes for the release

- Person to whom the information is to be released

When a resident, responsible party, or family member requests a medical record, make sure the person requesting the information is legally entitled to it. For example, the confused resident's adult daughter is designated as the durable power of attorney for healthcare. However, the son requests a copy of the medical record. He is not entitled to a copy of the record unless the daughter named the resident's healthcare proxy signs a record release.

When "all records" are requested, you must copy records from the open chart, permanent medical records file, unfiled thinnings, and all business office and billing records. If some records are from the hospital, physician, or other provider, you should copy them as part of the request. However, you are under no obligation to request or obtain records from other facilities for the purpose of furnishing them to the resident.

Make sure that both sides of two-sided forms are copied and collated together. You can staple them, but this may be very time consuming. This writer recommends stapling the MDSs and other long documents together individually. If these become separated, it is difficult or impossible to put them back together. Make sure the name and dates at the top and bottom are not cut off in copying. Make sure you do not cut off the sides of the MDS information. This is easily done because data is written close to the page margins.

In some facilities, chart forms are designed for binders that hold the records at the top. The forms are right side up on the front of the page and upside down on the back side. (This is called "top to tail.") Copy these records on single pages or make sure two-sided copies both face the same direction ("top to top"). Copy each telephone order and small-size laboratory report individually, or three to a page so they are legible. Avoid copying a page of documents filed with one order on top of the other. If this is the case, only the top document will be legible. There is no obligation to sort the record in a particular order, but avoid deliberately scrambling it.

When records have been requested, be honest and forthright. Avoid body language and demeanor that make it appear as if you are hiding something. Offer to interpret the information. An untrained observer comes up with many purported deficiencies because they do not understand the recordkeeping requirements. For example, the untrained reviewer may complain that there is "no nurse's note every shift," or "Doctor ordered MOM at bedtime PRN" and nurses seldom gave it, or a nurse gave it one day at 3:00 p.m. instead of HS. (The individual reviewing the record probably does not know the meaning of the PRN abbreviation.) Explaining these things to the reviewer may save you time, trouble, and grief over the long term.

A formal records request from a current or former resident, responsible party, or attorney usually means that someone is dissatisfied with care outcomes and they are considering a lawsuit. You may wish to notify your legal counsel if you have not already done so. You may also wish to review the record to determine whether care-related problems exist. However, you should avoid tampering with the record, removing pages, scrambling or rearranging the pages of the record. Some facilities try to tamper with flow sheets by filling in documentation gaps at this stage. Falsification causes the reader to question the credibility of the entire record. It is unlikely that filling in the boxes to show the resident had a shower three times a week will affect the plaintiff's allegations. In order to prove negligence, the plaintiff must have damages. Facilities do not always understand this, and focus on filling in documentation errors that are unrelated to the plaintiff's allegations.

Occasionally, the resident or responsible party will request and obtain a copy of the medical records involved before a lawsuit has been filed. This is usually done immediately after discharge. These records are provided to the attorney and are used as the basis for the initial review for merit screening. If a lawsuit is subsequently filed, the attorney will typically request a complete set of records from the facility. These records will be compared with the family's copy of the records to determine if the record was subsequently altered or if certain documents are missing. Discrepancies found during this review are used to damage the credibility and veracity of the medical record, the facility, and its personnel.

Clinical records service supervisor

Some states require facilities to designate a clinical records supervisor in writing. For example:

- The facility must designate in writing a clinical records supervisor who has the authority, responsibility, and accountability for the functions of the clinical records service. The clinical records supervisor must be (1) A registered health information administrator (RHIA) or registered health information technician (RHIT); or (2) An individual with experience appropriate to the scope and complexity of services performed as determined by the Texas Department of Human Services, and who receives consultation at a minimum of every 180 days from an (RHIA) or (RHIT).[18]

If a medical record is subpoenaed or requested by an attorney, the person responsible for medical records in your facility may be asked to sign an affidavit or declaration of authenticity attesting that the records provided are a true and complete copy of the medical records used and maintained by the facility during the usual course of business.

If another individual, service, or business has photocopied the records, the responsible person may also have to sign a declaration related to the photocopying. You will most likely need to sign the form in front of a notary public. The declaration or affidavit is governed by the laws of your state, but generally speaking, the person certifying the records does so under penalty of law, such as making a false statement in an official proceeding. The affidavit or declaration must be signed in a manner that, if falsely made, would subject the maker to criminal penalties under the laws where the declaration is signed. A party who subpoenas the records or enters the record into evidence must provide written notice of intention to all adverse parties, and must make the record and certification available for inspection sufficiently before their offer into evidence to give an adverse party a fair opportunity to challenge them.

If the subpoena names a specific person or position, such as the clinical records supervisor, he or she may be required to produce the records in person. If a subpoena states the custodian of records must appear and produce the records in person, then the facility may designate a person to make the appearance. Consult with your legal counsel if you are unsure. A subpoena is a legal document that should never be ignored, under penalty of law.

Requests for records related to litigation

Do not release records to an attorney, law firm, or other party until you have a properly signed release for production of the records, or a court ordered subpoena. A facility (Facility A) released a resident's medical records upon the request of an attorney who was defending another facility (Facility B) in a lawsuit filed by the resident. The resident subsequently filed suit against Facility A for releasing the records without proper consent. He sought damages for embarrassment and humiliation because the records were released to the opposing attorney. Facility B and its attorney sought to have the case dismissed, since the records were needed in a court proceeding.

The Court of Appeal of Louisiana upheld the suit, noting that it is a breach of medical confidentiality for a healthcare facility to release a resident's records before being served with a court subpoena or with a proper medical-records release executed by the resident. The court noted in its opinion that the attorney could have sought a court order compelling the resident to sign a release, or could have accessed the records by other means, such as issuing a subpoena. The fact that this was not done was a clear-cut violation of the resident's right to medical record confidentiality.[19]

Legal record reviews

Before a lawsuit is filed, the plaintiff attorney usually asks a legal nurse consultant or nursing expert to do a preliminary review of the medical records to determine whether the prospective lawsuit is meritorious. "The primary role of a legal nurse consultant (LNC) is to evaluate, analyze, and render informed opinions on the delivery of healthcare and its outcomes. For nearly 20 years, legal nurse consultants have acted as collaborators, strategists, and educators by offering support in medically related litigation and other medical-legal matters. An LNC is a registered nurse, unlike a paralegal or a legal assistant, and is a unique and valuable member of the litigation team. LNCs bring their health science education and clinical expertise to healthcare-related issues in the litigation process.

The practice of legal nurse consulting is performed in collaboration with attorneys and others involved in the legal process. The LNC's scope of practice does not include the independent practice of law. Legal nurse consulting is a specialty of nursing. Nursing education and experience set the LNC apart from other members of the legal team."[20]

The attorney will obtain information from the nurse about each of the four elements listed on the first page of this chapter to determine whether a potential lawsuit has merit. Although the attorney decides whether the case has merit, he or she does so after consultation with the nurse and other health professionals, as appropriate. The nurse reviewer will analyze the record for both strengths and weaknesses.

He or she will provide a preliminary report to the attorney, who will decide whether to file a lawsuit. If so, additional medical records may be requested, more comprehensive chart reviews will be done, and written chronologies and reports may be generated. The mechanics of this process are determined by attorney preference and strategy. The process is also limited by record availability. An incomplete record may produce inaccurate results, so having complete facility records is necessary. Although having a complete set of records (medical, billing, pharmacy, physician, hospital, long-term care, etc.) is ideal, reviewers may have to evaluate records in batches as they become available.

Some attorneys prefer verbal reporting only, whereas others require exhaustive chronologies and written reports. State laws apply to discovery of this nursing information. In general, all written information developed by a testifying expert must be disclosed to the other party. Written information developed by behind-the-scenes experts (called consulting experts) and legal nurse consultants are not disclosed unless an expert witness has reviewed the information and used it in formulating his or her opinion. Because of the disclosure rules, many attorneys do not share this information with testifying expert witnesses.

A record request is also a tip-off that the survey team may visit soon for a complaint investigation. Plaintiff attorneys often encourage disgruntled families to call the abuse and neglect reporting hotline. The results of the complaint survey may harm or help you if the case proceeds to trial, depending on the surveyors' findings. In any event, be prepared for visitors. If the resident was discharged a long time previously, the attorney may prepare a written report and attach parts of the medical record for the family to send to the state survey agency.

Record analysis

Each resident's medical record is a legal source of evidence of services provided by the facility, its physicians, and consultant personnel. The medical record is an objective source of care given and the resident's response. A thorough and concise medical record suggests that adequate care was given.[21] An inadequate, incomplete chart suggests inadequate care was given. Since the medical record represents the nucleus of the residents' care, a thorough record review is the core of any legal action. In a lawsuit, attorneys and others will review all facility records pertaining to the resident, including billing information. They will also review hospital records, physician office records, and records from other facilities in which the resident lived.

When the determination has been made to progress to a lawsuit, the attorney will retain licensed professionals who are experienced in the care given and documentation standards to review and analyze the medical records. These reviewers are usually physicians and/or nurses who are familiar with long-term care facility standards and documentation requirements. Like yourself, they have the education and experience to determine whether the applicable standards of care were met. The reviewer analyzes the record for information that is included as well as omissions in documentation.

In fact, omissions are often very important to the legal review. This may be as simple as a skip on a flow sheet, or as complex as checking each MDS for a five-year residency period to ensure all are present and were completed when indicated. The reviewer will read and compare information on the medical record with other data available, such as Medicaid and Medicare documentation, bills, ambulance, and hospital records. He or she is looking for consistencies and contradictions.

The record reviewer may sort the record so that like documents are together. Ideally, the record will be received in this order, but often it is not. Working from a sorted record saves expert time and money, and greatly improves accuracy because of the detailed nature of the review and large amount of cross checking necessary.

Each medical record reviewer has their own preference for chart order. Many sort the record in a manner similar to the open medical record, except that the various sections are arranged chronologically, by date, from oldest to most recent. Charts reviewed in this manner read like a book, and finding information is relatively simple. In a long-term care facility lawsuit, the reviewer usually reads every word of the nursing home record.
Always avoid the temptation to repair or alter a medical record. Provide it to the requesting party replete with skips and documentation problems. Checking for signs of alteration or falsification is a routine part of the record review. However, most reviewers will tell you they have never reviewed a mistake-free medical record.

The reviewer is not looking for a perfect record, isolated flow sheet skips or harmless documentation errors. He or she evaluates patterns of skips and errors and compares them with the injuries sustained by the resident. For example, in a given month, one would expect to find documentation of the resident's food consumption for at least 90 meals. In our example record, documentation omissions were made and only 60 meals were documented. If there was no weight loss or related nutritional problem, this is most likely a nonissue. However, if the resident experienced a significant weight loss during the month, you can expect the skips to be problematic as the lawsuit progresses.

The implication may be that the resident was not given 30 meals during the month. There appears to be a direct relationship between the documentation skips and the weight loss. However, the reviewer will also consider the skips in the context of the resident's diagnoses, physician orders, care plan, labs, dietitian notes, and other related information. The flow sheet will not stand on its own when drawing conclusions about resident injuries. Thus, the documentation skips are a small part of a much larger puzzle.

Minimum data sets

The minimum data sets (MDS) and care plans are especially important in long-term care lawsuits, related to evaluating resident improvement, declines, and overall nursing care. These documents are the foundation of the nursing process, as well as all resident care. The medical record reviewer will be addressing the resident holistically, and looking for patterns of excellent care, as well as poor care. The remainder of the record will be compared with the MDS for consistencies and inconsistencies. Accurate completion of the MDS is particularly important. If the facility misses an item that is a potential trigger, a care plan problem may be missed. If the facility states the resident is terminally ill and the decline was unavoidable, the reviewer will review the terminal illness section of the MDS. He or she will depend on the MDS to determine whether problems such as contractures were present on admission and compare these data with the time of discharge. Again, the MDS is reviewed in the context of the information elsewhere in the record. The data are not isolated. Putting it bluntly, the government has handed you a wealth of information to use in providing quality care for the residents. If the facility does not use it as intended, a legal reviewer may find a way to use the information to show the facility did not meet the applicable standards of care.

Care plans

The care plan is a source of great consternation for many facilities (Chapters 4 and 10). Each resident is unique and facility staff must maintain a commitment to individualized care that meets the resident's needs. The legal reviewer uses critical thinking and the nursing process when evaluating the care plan and comparing it with information on other parts of the record. He or she will try to determine whether the care plan provides a representative snapshot of the resident during his or her stay in the facility. The reviewer is not looking for a perfect care plan.

He or she may consider some care plan omissions significant and others insignificant. The concern here is whether the plan provides an overview of the resident's strengths and needs and whether the plan is used to drive the care provided by the facility. If the reviewer finds evidence of adequate care elsewhere on the record, a care plan omission is often considered a harmless documentation error. However, if the reviewer finds evidence of substandard care resulting in harm to the resident, care plan omissions suggest serious breaches of duty.

Facilities often have difficulty keeping care plans current. Having a temporary care plan form initiated at the time of admission is a helpful tool. Include obvious problems and potential problems. When the MDS and care plan are completed, incorporate the relevant information, then file the temporary plan.

A temporary plan may also be useful between care plan reviews. If a resident experiences a change in condition, injury, infection, or other problem, the nurse discovering the problem should add the information to the temporary plan of care. In this case, the temporary plan is used as a supplement to the full care plan. The temporary plan is updated when necessary, and filed when the condition is no longer problematic. Updating temporary care plans usually requires the knowledge of a nurse who works on the unit. A facility MDS nurse or care plan coordinator may not be immediately aware of incidental changes in each resident's condition that should be care planned.

The care plan is reviewed and updated quarterly and whenever a change in condition occurs. However, if a resident experiences a change in a high risk condition, such as a fall or pressure ulcer, it is a good idea to evaluate and update the plan of care immediately. Likewise, if a resident experiences recurrent problems, such as skin tears, falls, urinary infections, etc., the reviewer will evaluate how these are managed on the plan of care.

The plan should be adjusted when problems occur. If the resident has a fall prevention plan and experiences recurrent falls, the plan is ineffective. Change it immediately. Do not wait for the quarterly care conference! Even minor problems, such as recurrent skin tears warrant care plan adjustments. The reviewer will look to see if the plan was changed in a timely manner. He or she will look elsewhere in the record to determine whether the care listed on the plan was being delivered. Having a perfect written plan is purposeless.

The reviewer will use critical thinking and healthcare knowledge to determine whether the nursing process was used and the resident benefited from the plan adjustments and updates. He or she will also determine whether the resident's problems were unavoidable based on this review.

Physician orders

A legal record reviewer will read each physician order and telephone order on the medical record. A great deal of cross checking is done with physician orders to determine whether they were implemented, evaluated, and the physician notified of the resident's progress (or lack of progress), as necessary. Part of the chart audit involves cross-checking information from the nurses' notes, care plan, medication and treatment records to ensure facility response to resident problems was appropriate and timely, and that physician orders were implemented reasonably soon after a problem occurred. He or she will look for notification of the closest family member or other responsible party.

The reviewer will check to ensure follow-up monitoring was appropriate if the resident had a medical (or other) problem. Depending on the nature of the problem, the reviewer may audit additional records, such as laboratory reports and social service notes. The reviewer will also look for evidence of the physician's involvement in the plan of care. If the attending physician was not available to respond to a nurse's call, the reviewer will determine whether subsequent nursing action and notifications were appropriate.

If the nurse reviews a telephone order suggesting an incident, injury, or other problem, he or she will refer to the nurses' notes to find documentation of the problem, as well as follow-up care. A common problem is finding telephone orders for obvious problems with no corresponding nurses' note.

Falsifying telephone orders

Some nurses feel secure in knowing what various physicians commonly order in usual situations. They fill out telephone orders listing the physician's "usual" practices and preferences without actually contacting the physician. This is never a safe practice unless you are writing a telephone order to implement approved facility protocols, standing orders, or policies and procedures. If a medical record is involved in a lawsuit, the physician will most likely testify that he or she did not approve the nursing order. This exposes the nurse to potentially serious criminal penalties and adverse licensure action.

Reading back orders

One Joint Commission requirement for accredited facilities is that telephone and verbal orders must be "read back" to the person who originated the order for confirmation. Although most long-term care facilities are not Joint Commission accredited, this is still an important safety policy to consider and adopt. The readback requirement applies to all orders and "critical test results."

A "critical test result" is any lab or other diagnostic test, such as imaging studies and electrocardiograms ordered stat or returns with a panic value.

Readbacks of telephone and verbal orders

The readback rule applies whenever a nurse takes a telephone or verbal order. Simply repeating the order is not sufficient. According to the Joint Commission, the intent of the rule is for the nurse to receive and document the complete order, then read it back to the physician who gave the order.

Readbacks for critical test results

When reporting critical test results, the Joint Commission expects the facility to establish a procedure in which the physician (or other healthcare professional) "reads back" the critical test results to the person who reported them. Facility staff should request the "readback" whenever communicating critical test results verbally, including over the telephone.

Voice mail and electronic messages

The Joint Commission will not accept a voice mail or verbal electronic message for satisfying the readback requirement. They note that "most state laws require nurses and pharmacists to obtain the order directly from the prescriber or his or her agent." When the order is not received directly, the nurse (or pharmacist) must call the prescriber back to obtain the order directly, including a "readback."

Verification of readbacks

The Joint Commission requires verification of readbacks, but leaves the method to the facility. Some facilities have added "RB" to their accepted abbreviation list, denoting the order was "read back." The person receiving the order notes "RB" when he or she signs the verbal or telephone order. For example, the nurse writes the following on the order sheet:
"TO/Dr. Kritzberg/S. Lovewell, RN/RB/SL" This means: Nurse Lovewell received a telephone order ("TO") from Dr. Kritzberg, read it back ("RB") to him or her, and initialed the documentation ("SL").

Surveyors may ask how the facility tracks readback performance to ensure it is being done consistently. Many facilities are doing audits of phone and verbal orders each month. If compliance is less than a designated percentage (such as 95% of the orders comply, 5% do not), the facility should consider remedial action.

A medical-legal reviewer will also consider presence or absence of readback documentation when making determinations about the credibility and veracity of the medical record.

Progress notes

The physician must write a progress note each time he or she visits the resident. The physician must see the resident once every 30 days for the first 90 days, then every 60 days after that. After the initial visit, the physician may alternate face-to-face visits with a nurse practitioner, clinical nurse specialist, or physician assistant. The reviewer will determine whether physician visits were made in the specified time frame and whether the resident was also seen by a nurse practitioner or other professional. If so, he or she will look for evidence that the physician was managing the care.

The medical-legal review involves reading every detail of the physicians' progress notes. He or she will cross check information against nursing notes and other records, as appropriate. If the physician has ordered routine monitoring, such as vital signs and intake and output every shift or weights daily, the reviewer will look for evidence that this was done. If the physician writes an order such as, "Encourage fluids," the reviewer will look for evidence that this was added to the care plan and done consistently every shift.

Nurses do not have the authority to omit basic procedures ordered by the physician, or to pick and choose which physician orders they will follow. All physician orders must be followed and many warrant a care plan note or addition.

The reviewer will weigh and consider physician progress notes stating that certain declines were unavoidable. However, other factors must also be considered when determining whether a problem was unavoidable. The physician note is an important consideration, but is not taken at face value without additional supportive information about the problem.

The presence of a high-risk condition does not make certain problems inevitable. If a high-risk condition is noted, the chart reviewer will determine whether the facility has provided effective prevention and treatment of the condition, based upon consistently providing routine and individualized interventions.

A condition such as a pressure ulcer is determined to be "unavoidable" if the problem occurred despite the facility's best prevention efforts. This means the facility has identified and acted on the risk by taking steps to reduce or ameliorate risk factors, and providing preventive care. They have implemented interventions that are consistent with resident needs, goals, and recognized standards of practice. The facility must effectively and consistently monitor and evaluate the effectiveness of their interventions; and revise the approaches to care, when appropriate. If these things have not been done, the reviewer will most likely consider the skin breakdown or other problem to be avoidable with proper care.

Nursing notes

The nurse reviewer will read every nursing note in the record. Depending on the resident's outcome, he or she will evaluate various aspects of the care given. The nurse reviewer wants to know about the resident. He or she does not want to read several years worth of notes describing the care of a gastrostomy tube (such as, "G-tube patent.") You are caring for a person, not a tube! Make sure narrative documentation describes the resident and his or her condition. Normal observations, such as "G-tube patent" can be easily documented on a flow sheet.

Use the nursing notes to describe:

- Medical or behavior problems

- Discovery of or change in skin condition, such as skin tears and pressure ulcers

- Incidents and accidents such as falls

- Abnormal vital signs leading to focused system assessments

- Documentation of notifications made on the resident's behalf

Ongoing monitoring of abnormalities is important, as is the evaluation of the effectiveness of treatment. For example, if the resident has a URI, the reviewer may expect to find a note about lung sounds, nasal congestion, or cough. If the only entry states, "No side effects to antibiotic," there is no way to evaluate the resident's condition and corresponding nursing actions. If a reviewer finds a pattern of recurrent documentation of like problems (such as recurrent UTIs, falls, or skin tears) in the nurses' notes, he or she will look for recognition of high risk for this condition, and will review the care plan to determine whether the problem is being addressed. He or she will also determine whether illnesses were identified and monitored appropriately, in a timely manner.

Residents with high-risk conditions, changes in condition, or signs of acute illness require complete assessment and frequent monitoring. The assessment and implementation information must be thoroughly documented. If the chart ends up in court, the jury may not believe monitoring was appropriate unless it is documented. Verbal testimony indicating nurses checked the resident is viewed with suspicion in absence of proper documentation. Often, family members will contradict nursing testimony by stating that no one assessed the resident despite their pleas. If their testimony is consistent with the resident's outcome, jurors will likely accept it as the truth.

If a nurse documents numeric observations such as a resident's weight, appetite or bowel movement on the nurses' notes, you can expect the reviewer to cross check these data on the flow sheets. Finding contradictions, such as "Appetite 15%" in nursing notes and "100%" on the flow sheet is not uncommon. If the nurses' notes indicate the physician was called, the reviewer will check the telephone orders. If a medication or treatment was ordered, he or she will also check the appropriate flow sheet and care plan to determine if and when the order was implemented.

If the resident transferred from your facility to a hospital or another long-term care facility, you can expect the plaintiff attorney to request their records as well.

They may also subpoena transportation providers, such as the ambulance service. When a resident is transferred to the acute care hospital, the nurse reviewer will expect to find an assessment of the problem in the nursing notes, as well as the action taken, notifications, monitoring, and transfer. The reviewer will also compare, contrast, and evaluate the data on the transfer form, ambulance run sheet, and hospital admitting record to determine whether the information is consistent or contradictory. He or she will also compare the resident's condition on admission with documentation of the resident's condition upon discharge from the long-term care facility.

For example, a facility nurse documents the resident's foley is "draining clear amber urine." The ambulance run sheet notes the drainage bag is empty. The ER nurse notes "gross hematuria with mucous shreds and sediment in catheter drainage bag." Another typical example is the long-term care facility documenting a 1-centimeter Stage I ulcer on the coccyx, with the hospital documenting a malodorous 4-centimeter Stage IV ulcer in the same location. The records of the ambulance service and emergency department sometimes reflect poorly upon the long-term care facility.

When a resident is transferred to the hospital, labs are usually drawn on admission. The legal reviewer will study the laboratory reports to determine whether preventable abnormalities are present. He or she will review the time of the facility discharge note, ambulance arrival and departure, and ambulance arrival at the hospital, and time of emergency department or hospital admission to determine whether they are all within the same approximate time frame. Prolonged delays may be questioned.

Laboratory, x-ray, and related reports

The nurse reviewer will evaluate the laboratory reports. If the physician orders routine labs, such as a CBC monthly, the nurse will determine whether the labs were done as ordered. He or she will determine when the sample was drawn, and when the result was phoned or faxed to the facility. If the laboratory values are abnormal, he or she will try to determine whether facility personnel recognized and acted on the abnormality by making phone contact with the physician, notifying other professionals such as the dietitian, as appropriate, and updating the plan of care.

If the laboratory reports were not returned in a reasonable period of time, the reviewer will try to determine why. He or she will also look for evidence that the facility was aware that lab reports were missing, and action taken to rectify the problem. If the lab reports suggest correctable medical problems, he or she will also review the care plan. For example, the BUN value is elevated by two points suggesting early (mild) dehydration. Other values are normal.

The legal nurse consultant will look for facility recognition of the problem and prompt physician notification. Nursing observations, actions, and special monitoring should be listed on the care plan and implemented when appropriate, such as by adding I&O monitoring and placing an I&O flow sheet in the record.

Dietitian notes

The dietitian's assessment and notations are an important part of the medical-legal review. Many long-term care facility residents have problems related to nutrition and hydration. The dietitian also plays an important role in the management of various medical problems, such as diabetes and pressure ulcers.

The dietitian will document the resident's height and weight on admission. He or she will use these data to perform certain mathematical calculations, such as the resident's minimum daily caloric and fluid needs. The dietitian will review the available laboratory reports and may make recommendations for care (such as increasing fluids) or additional monitoring, such as repeating the hemoglobin and hematocrit in thirty days. He or she may also make nutritional recommendations, such as adding a vitamin or high-calorie nutritional supplement.

The dietitian will review the diet order and resident food consumption for appropriateness and adequacy, and may also make recommendations for changes in this area. Nursing personnel are expected to read the dietitian's documentation and consult the physician for a change in orders, when necessary. Omissions of this nature are often significant.

The medical legal reviewer will compare the dietitian's calculations of the resident's minimum fluid and caloric needs with the intake and output record, meal consumption record, weight records (including weights documented on the MDS.) He or she will review documentation of supplements and nourishments, and calculate caloric values of the products being given. The reviewer will determine whether the facility has been attentive to providing sufficient fluids and nutrients. If not, he or she will consider information on care plans, nursing notes, and other records to determine whether problems such as weight loss, malnutrition, and dehydration were avoidable.

A surprising number of tube-fed residents develop malnutrition and dehydration as a result of nursing failure to provide fluid and supplement solutions as ordered by the physician and dietitian. Documentation of care for residents with feeding tubes is often in good order, with no skips or apparent documentation problems. If the tube-fed resident experiences dehydration, malnutrition, or significant weight loss, the reviewer will probably question the credibility, integrity, and veracity of the documentation unless the resident has terminal cancer or another medical condition to account for the problem.

Other documentation

The medical-legal reviewer will read, review, compare, and contrast all other documents on the facility record, including flow sheets, therapy evaluations and notes, pharmacist notes (if any), social services, and activities records. These may or may not be important to the review, depending on the resident's medical problems and injuries alleged. They may also become important if they reflect problems or observations with no nursing follow-up.

Contradictions between these records and the MDS and nursing records may also be significant. The reviewer will check to see that these departments have provided consultation and participation to relevant resident problems. He or she will consider the care plan and flow sheets to determine whether care given is in keeping with the recommendations of therapists, the social worker, and other professionals, when indicated.

As you can see, the determination to go forward with a lawsuit is based on this initial review of the medical records. The facility has a very limited time frame in which to produce the records. Making sure that documentation is accurate and concise when the record is open and ongoing is the best protection you can provide. After the record has been closed, sorting it and putting it in facility-designated order will make it much easier to review. Once again, the facility is being evaluated based on external appearances. A complete, concise, accurate and organized medical record will help project a positive image of the facility, and reduce the risk that a lawsuit will proceed.

Theories of recovery

If a lawsuit is filed as a result of this record review, it will probably contain one or more of these theories of recovery:

- General negligence. (Allegations of negligent hiring, negligent supervision, negligent retention of staff and understaffing.)

- Aggregate (pattern) of poor care, including recurrent incidents and injuries, such as skin tears, pressure ulcers, falls, or fractures.

- Medical malpractice.

- Negligence Per Se (statutory violation of Omnibus Budget Reconciliation Act, state laws, and/or federal regulations).

- Breach of contract (breach of the admission agreement and care plan)

  - In assisted living facilities, this is breach of the service plan. Assisted living facilities have fewer regulations to provide substance to complaints alleging breach of the standard of care. For this reason, many lawsuits emphasize the importance of breach of contract and failure to have or follow the service plan.

- Failure to fulfill promises on marketing brochures and advertising materials, such as "24-hour nursing care provided." The facility does not provide 24-hour nursing care to each resident. A more appropriate statement may be, "Nursing personnel on duty 24 hours a day."

- The plaintiff may also approach "breach of contract" from the opposite direction. The facility also contracts with the state agency who administers the Medicaid program. As part of the contract with this agency, the facility pledges that it will comply with the agency's rules and regulations on a continual basis. The facility promises to correct all deficiencies in a timely manner. These provisions establish a cause of action for breach of contract in facilities with an ongoing history of relevant deficiencies.

The lawsuit may also request an award for punitive damages. A claim for punitive damages is appropriate if the facts of the case are considered egregious. In most states, the plaintiff must demonstrate gross, wanton, or willful misconduct to recover punitive damages.

Most lawsuits are filed in state court. Occasionally, long-term care cases are filed in federal court. The plaintiff is not required to file in federal court, even if he or she alleges a breach of federal laws. However, occasionally cases are filed in federal court for other reasons, such as circumventing state medical malpractice caps. Sometimes the charges result in criminal prosecution of individuals, if allegations of abuse and neglect are proven.

Threats to licensure

A single complaint against a nurse can trigger an investigation of the nurse's practice. The complaint can be filed by a resident, colleague, physician, or hospital administrator. As the agency responsible for regulating the practice of nursing in each state, the Board of Nursing has a duty to investigate all allegations. If the investigator agrees with the complainant that the nurse poses a clear and immediate danger to the public's health and safety, the board will take disciplinary action.

When the case and the medical record are reviewed by external reviewers (state department of public health surveyors, the Board of Nursing or the Board of Medicine, or a patient's attorney), there is the potential for action against your nursing license. There could be allegations that you breached your state Nurse Practice Act, that you did not meet the "just and prudent" nurse measure, or that your practice violated state, federal, or professional standards. All of these allegations will be analyzed to evaluate the nursing action in question, and in many cases, your defense lies in the clinical record and is based on your nursing documentation.

Pertinent medical records, human resource files, and copies of the organization's policies and procedures will all be reviewed. The Board of Nursing may also ask an independent nurse consultant to review your documentation to determine whether your actions were appropriate. If it finds that your actions were inappropriate, the board could approve any of the following disciplinary actions:

- Censure

- Letter of reprimand

- Probation (time defined)

- Suspension of license

- Revocation of license

Civil litigation

Residents have high expectations of their medical care. When we do not meet their expectations, their anger can turn into both allegations of negligence and professional negligence lawsuits. Malpractice cases regarding alleged nursing errors in long-term care facilities are increasingly making local and national headlines—and individual nurses are now being named to avoid statutory caps on payments. This strategy of naming an employee (nurse) as a direct defendant along with the employer (nursing home) relates to the legal view under the respondent superior, or "let the master answer," doctrine.

A negligence lawsuit is typically a civil case. The plaintiff relies on tort law, which includes negligence and professional negligence. A tort is a civil wrong for which the law allows the injured party to seek damages. Negligence is defined as conduct that falls below the standard established by law for the protection of others against unreasonable risk of harm. It includes the concept of "foreseeability"—in other words, that the harm that occurred could have been anticipated. For nurses, this is measured by "the ordinary, reasonable, and prudent nurse" standard.

For a nurse to be found negligent, the resident must prove the following:

- **Duty:** The resident must show that the nurse had a duty to the resident

- **Breach of duty:** The resident must define the appropriate standard of care and show that the nurse violated that standard

- **Causation or proximate cause:** The resident must prove that this breach of duty caused the injury

- **Damages or injuries:** The resident must prove that there are damages as a result of the breach or as a result of the nurse's negligent actions

So how does documentation tie into civil litigation? The resident's attorney will educate jurors as to the importance of documentation in the clinical record. They will inform jurors of why timely and accurate documentation is important and how it reflects good patient care. Therefore, jurors will view good recordkeeping as an indicator of quality care and poor documentation as an indicator of poor care. Poor nursing documentation will decrease the credibility of the nurse—even if the nurse maintains that the care was provided, the jurors will rely on the evidence in the clinical record.

State Nurse Practice Acts

The Standards of Nursing Practice clearly articulate what is expected of every practicing nurse. It is your responsibility to know your scope of practice in your state. Your state's Nurse Practice Act will define what is expected of you when providing nursing care. If you are in nursing management, you are evaluated for whether your management of resident care and your staff's practice reflects contemporary nursing practice.

Your first duty is to ensure that you understand your state Nurse Practice Act and that the staff nurses also know and understand it. One useful way to address this need is to have the risk manager or hospital attorney provide an annual inservice for your staff with case studies regarding the state practice act and documentation issues. You may consider having your nurse educators videotape this inservice so that it is available for all staff. An effective inservice with actual examples of litigation concerns demonstrating the significance of these issues often gets the staff's attention and also provides expert advice to the staff. You may want to consider giving this inservice at the same time that you are dealing with other mandatory inservice issues, such as fire safety and CPR, so that the staff become accustomed to this annual update and take responsibility for keeping themselves informed.

References

1. Texas Board of Nurse Examiners. (2006). Nurse Practice Act. Online. http://www.bne.state.tx.us. Accessed 02/11/06.
2. Better Documentation. (1992). Springhouse, Pa.: Springhouse Corp., 39.
3. Thomas v. Greenview Hosp., Inc., __ S.W. 3d __, 2004 WL 221198 (Ky. App., February 6, 2004).
4. Better Documentation. (1992). Springhouse, Pa.: Springhouse Corp., 39.

5. Morris, JN, Murphy, K., Nonemaker, S. (2002). Long-term care facility resident assessment instrument (RAI) user's manual. Des Moines. Briggs Corp.

6. Morris, JN, Murphy, K., Nonemaker, S. (2002). Long-term care facility resident assessment instrument (RAI) user's manual. Des Moines. Briggs Corp.

7. State Operations Manual. §483.75(j)(1) Laboratory Services.

8. U.S. Department of Health and Human Services (Eds). (1992). Pressure Ulcers in Adults: Prediction and Prevention. Rockville, MD. Agency for Health Care Policy and Research.

9. U.S. Department of Health and Human Services (Eds). (1992). Pressure Ulcers in Adults: Prediction and Prevention. Rockville, MD. Agency for Health Care Policy and Research.

10. U.S. Department of Health and Human Services (Eds). (1994). Pressure Ulcer Treatment. Rockville, MD. Agency for Health Care Policy and Research.

11. Hess, Cathy Thomas. (1998). Nurse's Clinical Guide Wound Care. Springhouse, PA. Springhouse Corporation.

12. Tscheschlog, B. et al (Eds). (1995). Mastering documentation. Pennsylvania, Springhouse. Springhouse Corporation.

13. State Operations Manual. §483.10(b)(2)

14. Chart Smart: The A-to-Z guide to better nursing documentation. (2001). Springhouse, Pa.: Springhouse Corp., ix, 203, 301.

15. Richards, M. (2001). Documentation - a vital and essential element of the nursing process. Survey Savvy. Des Moines, Briggs Corporation.

16. Morris, J.N., Murphy, K., Nonemaker, S. (2002). Long-term care facility resident assessment instrument (RAI) user's manual. DesMoines. Briggs Corp.

17. State Operations Manual. §483.10(b)(2)

18. Texas Administrative Code. §19.1913.

19. Sanders vs. Spector, 673 So. 2d 1176 (La. App., 1996).

20. American Association of Legal Nurse Consultants. (1999). Getting started in legal nurse consulting: An introduction to the specialty, second edition. Chicago. American Association of Legal Nurse Consultants.

21. This statement is made assuming that the reviewer is analyzing the original open or closed medical record; not a record that was subsequently altered or corrected.

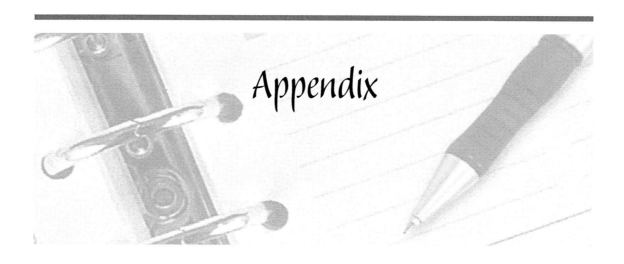

Appendix

FIGURE A.1

AFFIDAVIT TO ACCOMPANY MEDICAL RECORDS

I_____(custodian of records of resident)_____
do hereby declare:

I am the duly authorized custodian of the medical records of _____, or other
qualified witness with authority to certify the records.

2. [ ] The records you seek may contain information regarding alcohol or drug abuse records, the results
of a blood test for HIV, or information regarding certain psychiatric, mental health, or developmental
disabilities. This information, if it exists, may be protected by special state and federal laws and
cannot be released without specific written authorization by the resident or pursuant to other
procedures established by law. A subpoena or general authorization for release of medical records
is not sufficient.

[ ] I do not have the records described in the subpoena.

[ ] These medical records are true copies of all the records in my possession described in the subpoena
which are allowed by law to be released.

[ ] The records described in the subpoena and authorized by law to be released were delivered to
_____ on _____ (date)

I declare under penalty of perjury that the above statements are true and correct and that this declaration
was made at _____, on _____ (date)

Signed:_____
　　　　　　　　　　　　　Affiant

Print name: _____ Phone _____

　　　SUBSCRIBED AND SWORN TO BEFORE ME, _____, on this day,
personally appeared _____, known to me to be the person whose name is subscribed
to the foregoing instrument and acknowledge to me that he/she executed the same for the purpose and
consideration therein expressed.

　　　Given under my hand and seal of office this _____ day of _____.
　　　Signature of Notary: _____
　　　Notary Public in and for The State of _____
　　　My Commission Expires On: _____

FIGURE A.2

DOCUMENTATION FORMATS AND SYSTEMS

Many different documentation formats are used. In most long-term care facilities, medications, treatments, and ADLs are recorded on flow sheets. The caregiver initials a box to validate that care was given. Other common formats are the *narrative format*, and *acronym documentation*. The narrative format is written in complete or abbreviated sentences, and is preferred by most nurses. Many therapists prefer to document in the acronym and POMR formats because they can be readily used to describe neuromuscular problems. The acronym and POMR formats probably provide a higher level of legal protection because they force use of the nursing process for completing the documentation requirements. In a narrative charting system, notes may lack substance or are meaningless, such as "good day," "status quo," "up and about," or "usual day."

The format used should be based on the setting and to some extent, resident acuity. However, regardless of the format selected, nurses must always chart clinically significant observations, changes in the residents' conditions, and nursing response. To document changes, the chart must contain a reasonably accurate picture of the resident's baseline status, from which the changes may be measured.

Narrative documentation

Narrative documentation is chronological and describes the resident's condition and care in story book format. Assessment is an important part of this format. Most facilities chart narrative notes by writing complete sentences on lined pages. Occasionally, a facility uses a two or three-column approach to organize information. For example, a separate column may be used for vital signs, PRN medications, treatments, nursing observations, and related comments.

Nurses must make sure that narrative charting is legible and signed by each writer. Narrative notes may be supplemented with additional information, such as flow sheets. This type of documentation is seen in many lawsuits because it is commonly used in long-term care. Medical legal reviewers commonly identify problems with narrative charting, such as:

- incomplete documentation

- subjective information

- lack of descriptive narrative notes for a change in condition

- inability to verify appropriate use of the nursing process based on the record review

Some skilled nursing units use a combination of narrative and flow sheet charting. A new page is put into the nurses' notes every 24 hours. When using a 24-hour flow sheet to document care, such as on a skilled unit, the narrative notes should document the same 24-hour period. Half the form is general assessment information, with a box for each shift. Nurses check off each box, as appropriate. Variations from normal require a narrative note. This is a narrative charting format. It does not meet the criteria for Charting By Exception, even though it is similar to this method of documentation.

DOCUMENTATION FORMATS AND SYSTEMS (CONT.)

Focus charting

Focus charting was developed to cause nurses to view the resident in a positive light rather than the negative perspective commonly seen in documentation. The nurse must identify a focus of the documentation based on a change in condition, abnormal assessment data, or resident concerns. This system employs a three-column approach. Some facilities call this type of documentation DAR charting because of the acronyms described below:

- Data—The objective or subjective information supporting the focus identified by the nurse or describing nursing assessment and observations when a change in condition or significant event or treatment occurs.

- Action—This denotes any immediate or future nursing actions for the data listed, based on the nurse's evaluation of the resident's condition.

- Response—This section is used to describe the resident's response to medical and nursing care related to the identified problem.

An example of the format that is typically used for documentation is seen in Figure 1.

Figure 1   *Focus Charting Format*

Information	Date / Time	Focus	Progress (Narrative) Notes
Data:			
Action:			
Response:			

Acronym formats

Various acronyms are used to describe documentation requirements. Acronym documentation falls into the POMR category, described above. The acronyms ensure documentation of important observation and legal facts, such as assessment, actions and outcomes.

The SOAP format and related documentation

SOAP is an abbreviation for the categories that must be documented with each entry. Facilities using this format cannot usually pick and choose categories for each documentation. All entries include a statement for each category. For example:

- S means *subjective*. Symptoms are subjective findings, so they are described in this section.

DOCUMENTATION FORMATS AND SYSTEMS (CONT.)

This information is provided by the resident, family member, or another caregiver, such as a nursing assistant.

- O means *objective*. This information is based on direct observations by the nurse, including functional ability and signs of the resident's condition.

- A stands for *assessment*. Remember, only an RN can assess the residents. However, nursing assistants and practical/vocational nurses can collect and contribute data to the overall RN assessment. In some facilities, practical and vocational nurses call this category *analysis* because they cannot legally assess the resident. They write their analysis of the situation here.

- P stands for *plan*. The plan describes nursing care and treatment information. In this system, you will document the plan related to the problem described in each note. In some situations, documenting that you will continue using the same approaches to care may be appropriate, or that you will notify another professional of a problem.

Some facilities use the acronym SOAPIE to describe their documentation system. In this system, Implementation (nursing actions or interventions) and Evaluation (resident response to the plan of care for the item being documented) have been added. SOAPIER is another acronym used for documentation. In this system, an R is added to the last component to describe the Revision of the care plan, if any. When using a variation of the SOAP system,

the nurse should address each item of the word. Avoid skipping letters. Documentation may be a combination of complete and incomplete sentences and phrases.

The APIE format

APIE is a newer documentation system in which the nurse describes each element of the nursing process. This acronym means:

- A is resident *assessment*
- P stands for the *plan of care* for the problem (assessment) being documented
- I stands for *implementation* of the plan, in which the nurse writes a brief description of how the plan was implemented
- E is *evaluation* of the plan of care

In this method, documentation is condensed into fewer statements by combining subjective and objective data into the *Assessment* section and combining nursing actions and resident outcomes into the plan of care component. Like the SOAP system, all letters must be addressed. Documentation may be a combination of complete and incomplete sentences and phrases.

The PIE format

PIE is an acronym that describes problems, intervention and evaluation of the care rendered. In this system, a 24-hour flow sheet is used in addition to nurses' notes. The narrative notes are usually made only when the resident has a problem or abnormality. Each problem is assigned a number by the nurse. The narrative notes are usually written as numbered problem statements in which the formal nursing

DOCUMENTATION FORMATS AND SYSTEMS (CONT.)

diagnosis is listed as the problem. In this system:

- P denotes a problem statement (nursing diagnosis)
- I is the nursing intervention (care plan) for the problem
- E stands for the evaluation of the intervention or nursing action

Exception documentation

Exception documentation is done primarily through the use of two formal documentation systems:

- Charting by exception (CBE)

- Care mapping (may also be called concept mapping, critical pathways, variance analysis, and care analysis)

To be effective, these systems depend on a high degree of critical thinking and application of sound nursing judgment. Consistency between staff is a key to success when using exception systems. All nurses must document in the same manner. If some nurses complete their documentation in narrative and others use the exception format, there is a high probability that communication will be muddled or break down entirely. Some facilities have had problems with denials from Medicaid, Medicare, and insurance payments when exception documentation has been used. Narrative documentation is done only if assessment findings or care deviate from normals or standards of care established by the facility. In these systems, assessments are very thorough. A checklist is used to document normal findings. Narrative notes are used

to document abnormalities in the resident's condition or deviations from standards of care. These methods of documentation are not appropriate unless policies, procedures, and written standards of care exist and are regularly inserviced and used in the facility. The policies and procedures must be very explicit and state something like, "all standards of care have been met with a normal or expected response unless otherwise documented."

Charting by exception (CBE) documentation

This is a formal documentation system in which only significant findings, abnormalities, and exceptions to normal values are charted. The method of documenting is abbreviated, but the substance of the documentation is not deficient. This system is commonly employed for electronic documentation. A 24-hour flow sheet is used in addition to nurses' notes. At the time of the assessment, the nurse will check the various normal values on the assessment flow sheet. He or she will record an asterisk (*) if the resident has an abnormality, or a standard of care was not implemented. The nurse must write a narrative explanatory note to correspond with each asterisk.

- If your facility uses a charting by exception (CBE) format, use only exceptions to normal or expected observations. Describe abnormal findings and nursing action in a narrative note. Notify others as appropriate, and document notifications. Make sure the flow sheets you use accurately portray the resident and care given. Anytime the potential for unclear, inaccurate documentation exists, write the information in a narrative note.[1]

DOCUMENTATION FORMATS AND SYSTEMS (CONT.)

- Documentation tools for a CBE system should include the normal parameters for each system. Use the tools and normal parameters to document assessments and observations, as well as other pertinent data (i.e., vital signs, blood sugars, meal consumption, and intake and output). Be familiar with your facility CBE policies and procedures and follow them.

FACT documentation system

This is another common method used for electronic documentation. It is similar to CBE documentation. This method is believed to reduce repetition, prevent documentation of irrelevant information, and save time. This system uses flow sheets extensively. Unlike the acronym systems above, FACT does not list the various components of the chart entries. Typical documentation forms and flow sheets are:

- *Assessment and action*—documents ongoing assessments and corresponding nursing actions

  - Normal assessment findings for each anatomic system are often listed on the form with common, planned nursing interventions and actions. You must individualize the flow sheet to meet the resident's needs.

- *Frequent assessment*—the form on which you document vital signs and other assessments that must be done regularly, such as pain assessment or neurological checks

- *Progress notes*—space for narrative notes about resident progress and significant events or changes

in condition. The DAR method (described above in focus charting) is used for narrative notes.

Care mapping, concept mapping, and critical pathways

This type of documentation is popular in managed care environments, but the system follows the medical model of care and is not commonly used in traditional long-term care facilities. Pathways or maps are used for documenting and monitoring care. These forms are usually printed in advance and list the plan of care for various medical diagnoses and problems. The nurse personalizes the care map by checking boxes or writing approaches in longhand, such as diet, medications, activities, and treatments. The goal for this documentation system is to ensure the resident progresses according to the pathway. Deviations from the pathway are always a cause for concern and further investigation.

Care that progresses according to the pathway meets applicable standards for the diagnosis and is always cost effective. Variances and complications are often more expensive. Facilities that use care maps and pathways usually emphasize the provision of high quality, cost-effective care. Facilities encourage nursing personnel to strive to find new ways of providing care more efficiently and effectively without compromising quality. Doing this also reduces cost and increases the profit margin.

Reference

1. Smith, L.S. (2002). How to chart by exception. *Nursing*, 32(9), 30.

FIGURE A.3

EXAMPLE DISCLAIMERS FOR FAX AND EMAIL DATA TRANSMISSIONS

The information contained in this message is information protected medical information. It is intended only for the use of the individual named above and the privileges are not waived by virtue of this having been sent by electronic mail (or fax/facsimile). If the person actually receiving this message or any other reader is not the named recipient or the employee or agent responsible to deliver it to the named recipient, any use, forwarding, dissemination, distribution, or copying of the communication is strictly prohibited. If you have received this communication in error, please immediately notify us by telephone at (000) 000-0000. We will reimburse your costs to return the original message to us. Thank you.

The information contained in this message is information protected medical information. It is intended only for the use of the individual named above and the privileges are not waived by virtue of this having been sent by electronic mail (or fax/facsimile). If the person actually receiving this message or any other reader is not the named recipient or the employee or agent responsible to deliver it to the named recipient, any use, forwarding, dissemination, distribution, or copying of the communication is strictly prohibited. If you have received this message in error, do not read it. Please immediately notify the sender that you have received this communication in error. Then delete the information from your computer. (OR destroy information received by facsimile by shredding.) Thank you.

The information contained in the message is legally privileged, confidential information. If you are not the intended recipient, you are hereby notified that any use, dissemination, distribution, or copying of this message is strictly prohibited. Thank you.

Confidentiality Notice/disclaimer

The information contained in this email transmission is confidential and intended only for the use of the individual or entity named above. If you have received this transmission in error, please notify by email, and immediately delete the file/transmission from your computer. Thank you.

Confidentiality Notice: This email message, including any attachments, is for the sole use of the intended recipient(s) and may contain confidential and privileged information. Any unauthorized review, use, disclosure or distribution is prohibited. If you are not the intended recipient, please contact the sender by reply email and destroy all copies of the original message. Thank you.

EXAMPLE DISCLAIMERS FOR FAX AND EMAIL DATA TRANSMISSIONS (CONT.)

In accordance with the HIPAA (Health Insurance Portability & Accountability Act), this transmission contains protected health information for the sole use of the intended recipient. Any information is for the sole use of the intended recipient and any unauthorized use, disclosure, dissemination, distribution or copying of this information is prohibited. If you have received this in error, please notify us promptly. Thank you.

The information contained within this communication is privileged and confidential. In accordance with the HIPAA (Health Insurance Portability & Accountability Act), this email (OR attachment, OR facsimile) contains protected health information and for the sole use of the intended recipient's. Any unauthorized use, disclosure, dissemination, or copying of this information is strictly prohibited. If you receive this in error, do not read it. Please immediately notify to the sender that you have received this communication in error. Then delete the information from your computer. (OR destroy information received by facsimile by shredding.) Thank you.

***********CONFIDENTIALITY DISCLAIMER***************

The contents of this message may be privileged and confidential. Therefore, if this message has been received in error, please delete it without reading it. Your receipt of this message is not Intended to waive any applicable privilege. Please do not disseminate or distribute this message in any manner without the permission of the author. I expressly forbid the forwarding of any of email communications or facsimile transmissions to others unless written permission is obtained first. Thank you.

This e-mail is covered by the Electronic Communication Privacy Act, 18 U.S. C. 2510-2521 and is legally privileged. The information contained in this e-mail is intended only for use of the individual or entity named above. If the reader of this message is not the intended recipient, or the employee or agent responsible to deliver it to the intended recipient, you are hereby notified that any dissemination, distribution or copying of this communication is strictly prohibited. If you have received this communication in error, please immediately notify us by reply email or telephone (XXX-XXX-XXXX), and destroy the original message. The information is this transmission may contain privileged information that is protected under the Health Insurance Privacy Portability Act. Any use of this information against the act is strictly prohibited. Thank you.

EXAMPLE DISCLAIMERS FOR FAX AND EMAIL DATA TRANSMISSIONS (CONT.)

CONFIDENTIALITY DISCLAIMER: This message is confidential, intended only for the named recipient(s), and may contain information that is privileged or exempt from disclosure under applicable law. In accordance with HIPAA (Health Insurance Portability & Accountability Act), this E-mail/attachment may contain protected health information which is intended for the sole use of the intended recipient(s). Any unauthorized use, disclosure, dissemination, or copying of any information herein is prohibited. If you have received this e-mail/attachment in error, please notify the sender immediately and delete the information from your system. Thank you.

CONFIDENTIALITY DISCLAIMER: This email (fax/facsimile) and any files transmitted with it may contain confidential and/or proprietary information in the possession of __(NAME)__, and is intended only for the individual or entity to whom addressed. This email (Fax/Facsimile) may contain information that is held to be privileged, confidential and exempt from disclosure under applicable law. If the reader of this message is not the intended recipient, you are hereby notified that any unauthorized access, dissemination, distribution or copying of any information from this email is strictly prohibited, and may subject you to criminal and/or civil liability. If you have received this email (fax/facsimile) in error, please notify the sender by reply email (fax/facsimile) and then delete this email and its attachments from your computer (OR destroy the facsimile copy). Thank you.

Disclaimers cumulated with assistance from legal nurse consultants, attorneys, and other professional members of the Medical_Legal_Consultants and LNC Exchange listservs.

The information in this electronic mail message and any attachments is confidential and may be legally privileged. It is intended solely for the addressee(s). Access to this electronic mail message and any attachments by anyone else, is unauthorized. If you are not the intended recipient, any disclosure, copying, distribution, or any action taken, or omitted to be taken in reliance on it is prohibited and may be unlawful.

"The sender believes that this E-mail and any attachments were free of any virus, worm, Trojan horse, and/or malicious code when sent. This message and its attachments could have been infected during transmission. By reading the message and opening any attachments, the recipient accepts full responsibility for taking protective and remedial action

EXAMPLE DISCLAIMERS FOR FAX AND EMAIL DATA TRANSMISSIONS (CONT.)

about viruses and other defects. __(NAME)__ is not liable for any loss or damage arising in any way rom this message or its attachments."

If you are not the intended recipient, please promptly delete this message and notify the sender of the delivery error by e-mail or you may notify _____@_____ of the error.

DISCLAIMER: The information in this message and any attachment(s) is confidential and may be legally privileged. If you are not the intended recipient, please destroy this message, delete any copies held on your system and notify the sender immediately. You should not retain, copy or use this email for any purpose, nor disclose all or any part of its content to any other person.

Disclaimers cumulated with assistance from legal nurse consultants, attorneys, and other professional members of the Medical_Legal_Consultants and LNC Exchange listservs.

FIGURE A.4

AUTHORIZATION FOR RELEASE OF INFORMATION

Resident Information:

_____

(PRINT name of resident)   DOB   SS#

Information to be released from:

_____

Name of designated Facility or Provider

_____

Address

I request and authorize the above name facility or provider to release health care information of the patient named above to:

_____

Name of designated recipient

_____

Address

_____

City, State, Zip   Phone Number

Information to be Released

☐ The most recent 2 years of pertinent information (chart notes, labs, x-rays, and special tests)

☐ All medical records

☐ All Medical Billing Records

☐ Specific Information (Please Specify): _____

Purpose for which disclosure is being made: (Please check one of the following)

☐ Attorney   ☐ Insurance   ☐ Doctor   ☐ Personal

Resident Authorization:
I understand that my express consent is required to release any health care information relating to testing/diagnosis, and/or treatment for HIV (AIDS Virus), sexually transmitted diseases, psychiatric disorders/mental health, or drug and/or alcohol use. If I have been tested diagnosed, or treated for HIV (AIDS Virus), sexually transmitted diseases, psychiatric disorders/mental health, or drug and/or alcohol use, you are specifically authorized to release all health care information relating to such diagnosis, testing or treatment.

My Rights:
I understand I do not have to sign this authorization in order to obtain health care benefits (treatment, payment or enrollment). I may revoke this authorization in writing. To view the process for revoking this authorization, please read the Privacy Notice to patients posted at the facility where your information is being released. I understand that once the health information I have authorized to be disclosed reaches the noted recipient, that person or organization may re-disclose it, at which time it may no longer be protected under Privacy laws.

Reasonable Fee
State law provides that a health care provider may charge a reasonable fee.

_____   _____

Signature of Resident or Resident's Authorized Representative   Date Signed

This Authorization will expire 90 days from the date signed

FIGURE A.5

Authorization for Use or Disclosure of Protected Health Information

**INDIVIDUAL AUTHORIZATION FOR USE OR DISCLOSURE
PROTECTED HEALTH INFORMATION**

Section 1:

I hereby request and authorize the use or disclosure of my protected health information (PHI) as described below.

Resident Name   Resident Date of Birth   Resident SS#

_____   _____   _____

Resident Address   City, State & Zip Code   Resident Phone #

_____

The individual(s) or entity(ies) authorized to disclose the protected health information is/are:
Doctor:_____
Carrier: _____
Hospital: _____
Lab: _____
Other: _____

Section 2:

The individual(s) or entity(ies) authorized to receive the protected health information is/are:

_____

Section 3:

The types of protected health information that may be disclosed includes: (Check all that apply, and specify from [date] to [date] if you wish to limit by dates).
_____ Name and contact information only
_____ Name and contact information, diagnosis and treatment. Specific dates of illnesses or injuries:
_____ All medical records without restriction
_____ Complete medical records.
_____ Billing records. Dates: _____
_____Agreements and consents. Dates: _____

Authorization for Use or Disclosure of Protected Health Information

Pre- and post-op and surgery records. Specific surgeries or records? _____

Claims records, claims status, and resident management records.
Other: _____

Note: The protected health information disclosed to the entity you listed above may include information on chronic diseases, behavioral health conditions, including alcohol or substance abuse, communicable diseases, including HIV/AIDS, and/or genetic marker information.

Section 4:

The purpose for which the disclosure may be made is: (Check only one.)
_____ At the request of the individual.
_____ Other(s):_____

_____

_____

Section 5:

This authorization will be in force and effect until: (Check one.)
[Specify Date]:_____

If neither of above items are checked or completed, this Authorization will expire in one year from the date this Authorization is signed.

You have the right to revoke this Authorization at any time, by sending written notice to the individual or entity you listed above in Section 2. However, if you revoke this Authorization after protected health information has been disclosed, the disclosing entity will not be able to take back the information previously disclosed.

I hereby request and authorize the use or disclosure of my protected health information (PHI) as described above. I understand that if the organization authorized to receive the information is not a health plan or health care provider, the released information may no longer be protected by federal privacy regulations.

_____   _____

Signature of resident or legal representative, if applicable   Date

_____   _____

Print name of resident or legal representative*   Relationship to resident

*If this Authorization is being signed by the legal representative of the individual to whom the protected health information pertains, you must furnish a copy of the power of attorney or other relevant document designating you as the legal representative.

Authorization to Release Medical Information Form

Name: _____

Dates of treatment: _____

This is a request and authorizes all physicians, hospitals and medical attendants to furnish my complete and entire medical record of my treatment, diagnosis and tests including but not limited to: all medical reports and records, nurses' notes, x-rays, laboratory data, and all other information to me at the address provided below. This request and authority includes examination of originals of hospital records, admission and discharge records, X-rays, slides, and all other data, information and materials related to my treatment, including medical reports and opinions, and all lab data, with no exceptions. Please include a copy of each and every page of the medical record including but not limited to all notes written and dictated by physicians, consultants, nurses, and other health care providers. All previous authorizations are canceled, except those that permit release of information to facilitate payment of outstanding bills by any health insurance carrier. Please do not permit anyone else to review or inspect my records.

Dated:_____

Name_____

Signature_____

Address_____

City, State, Zip_____

FIGURE A.6

Inservice education

Devote time and effort to your inservice program. Many facilities conduct inservice on payday, an hour before handing out checks. Employees who are off-duty come in, often with children in tow. The inservice consists of a lecture or videotape. The same tapes are used repeatedly, so long-term staff usually have them memorized. This atmosphere is not conducive to learning.

Inservice education and regular staff communication meetings are important! Devote the effort to them that they deserve. Invite guest speakers for appropriate subject matter. Plan your inservices well, and vary your teaching methods. Examples of teaching methods and activities are

- Lecture—presents facts in a logical and direct manner. This is the most common teaching style, and is useful for large groups. However, it has several major drawbacks. The communication is one-way, the audience is passive, and visual learners may have difficulty grasping the concepts. Make sure the introduction is clear. Summarize at the end. Use examples and anecdotes liberally, and ask questions to stimulate critical thinking.

- Lecture with discussion is similar to a lecture, but is more participatory. In practice, students seldom interrupt to ask questions. However, using this format encourages student participation to question, clarify, and challenge the information. It is most effective when discussion questions are prepared in advance. The length of time available may adversely affect discussion quality and results.

- Group discussion is a means of blending and merging experiences and ideas from the entire group. This method is most effective when used after a presentation, film, or activity that requires further analysis. Guide the discussion with planning, questions, and directions related to the subject matter.

- Small-group discussion is effective in time-limited situations. For maximum effectiveness, the instructor should prepare questions for the group to answer. Participants learn teamwork. Small-group activities usually reach participants who are self-conscious and non-participatory in large groups.

- A panel is a group of experts in the subject matter. Experts are given a designated period of time to present their opinions. It is especially effective when the subject is controversial.

- Brainstorming is a participatory activity that is excellent to use when planning for change. This method encourages critical thinking and new ideas. Group members draw on each other's collective knowledge and experience, and participants learn teamwork. It is most effective when done in small groups, with a designated time limitation. At the end of the session, one group member summarizes group findings and recommendations for the class.

- Demonstration/Return Demonstration is a useful activity for teaching a new skill or learning to operate new equipment. Lecture

INSERVICE EDUCATION (CONT.)

and demonstrate the skill to the group. Break the large group down into smaller groups, and allow time for practice. Rotate among the groups while students are practicing. Single students out for praise. Avoid criticizing in public. After students have had an opportunity to practice, verify their competency in the skill.

- **Audiovisuals,** such as videotapes, DVDs, and other media such as Power Point slides, are entertaining, and excellent for visual learners. They are best used to reinforce lecture, demonstration, and reading material. An audiovisual as the sole teaching method may be ineffective. You can enhance student learning with a pre- and post-test, as well as prepared questions and activities for discussion after viewing the tape. When creating Power Point presentations, avoid using red and green together on a slide, because color blind students will have difficulty telling these colors apart.

- **Case studies** provide an excellent means for exploring complex issues. These activities help students develop critical thinking, analytic, and problem-solving skills. Make sure the case study is defined. For maximum effectiveness, students must have adequate background information and understand the relevance of the situation.

- **Role playing** provides an opportunity to learn by assuming the role of someone else and acknowledging his or her point of view.

This activity provides the opportunity to practice skills. However, some individuals may be self-conscious or uncomfortable in front of a group. Give clear instructions, define the problem or situation, and clearly state your expectations before beginning.

- **Reporting sessions** are an opportunity for class discussion or critique of role play, case studies, and small group activities. Prepare discussion questions and other activities in advance, and designate small groups for presentations.

- **Analogies** are useful when teaching new or difficult problems. Examples of this type of activity are to make comparisons between the cell and a factory, the eye with a camera, or the heart with a pump.

- **Worksheets and surveys** are intermittently useful. Students complete these activities independently in class. Their responses may be shared with the group.

- An **index card exercise** is useful for creating tools for future study. Give each student a stack of index cards. Instruct them to write down the important points and highlights of your lecture on each card. At the end of the session, collect the cards. File them in a common area where they can be reviewed as needed for future study.

- **Guest speakers** provide expertise on a variety of topics. They break monotony, and are use-

INSERVICE EDUCATION (CONT.)

ful in eliminating stereotypes and personalizing the subject matter. The instructor must plan the session, and contact and coordinate speakers. Make sure that the guest instructor understands the students' learning level and does not present material above or below that level.

- **Values-clarification activities** enable students to discuss values and beliefs in a safe environment. However, this activity may be threatening to self-conscious students. Structure the activity and prepare discussion questions. Moderate the discussion to keep things moving.

- **Assessing or evaluating** involves applying critical thinking skills based on available evidence or information. Teaching students to evaluate situations before reacting helps them learn to set priorities and develop good judgment. Students may answer questions based on patient care situations individually, as a group activity, or as a written assignment.

- **Right or Wrong** is an activity that may be done by showing pictures or slides or photos of problems and unacceptable conditions and having students identify them as a group. You can make the activity more participatory by preparing an area of the classroom with unacceptable conditions before students arrive. For example, set up a resident unit. Place a bottle of chemicals or denture cleaning tablets on the table. Place linen on the floor, or the urinal on a food tray. The objective is to create both obvious and subtle (realistic) conditions. Tell students the number of incorrect conditions. Have them write down as many as they can. Discuss them with the group, then relate the scenario to facility operations.

- **Games** are a fun, participatory method of learning. Create activities such as Safety BINGO, or model your games after television shows such as Jeopardy and Survivor. A surprising amount of learning takes place while your students are having fun.

FIGURE A.7

General Employee Orientation Inventory	Name: _____ Date Hired: _____

Curriculum	Date	Instructor Initials
A. Facility		
1. Purpose/Organization of the facility	_____	_____
a. function of a long-term care facility	_____	_____
b. tour facility	_____	_____
c. identify all departments and describe their functions	_____	_____
2. Philosophy of care	_____	_____
3. Chain of command	_____	_____
4. When/how to contact/notify administrator, supervisor, or department head on call	_____	_____
B. Personnel		
1. Employee job description/responsibilities	_____	_____
2. Operational policies and procedures	_____	_____
3. Personnel policies	_____	_____
a. working hours and schedules	_____	_____
b. holidays	_____	_____
c. sickness, vacation, leave	_____	_____
d. routine performance evaluations	_____	_____
e. verification of employee skills	_____	_____
f. verification of license, certification, credentials	_____	_____
g. criminal history check	_____	_____
h. random drug screening	_____	_____
i. pay schedule	_____	_____
j. other requirements and benefits	_____	_____
k. psychological and social needs of staff	_____	_____
4. Expectations/obligations of employees	_____	_____
a. keep facility informed of contact information	_____	_____
i. address	_____	_____
ii. telephone number	_____	_____
b. personal grooming/hygiene	_____	_____
i. daily bath, personal cleanliness	_____	_____
ii. clean clothing	_____	_____
iii. deodorant	_____	_____
iv. hair care, hair clean, long hair worn back or up, short/neat facial hair (males)	_____	_____
c. hands and fingernails	_____	_____
i. direct caregivers, dietary - nails no longer than 1/4 inch from tip of finger	_____	_____
ii. direct caregivers, dietary - no acrylic or sculpted nails	_____	_____
iii. direct caregivers, dietary - clear nail polish only	_____	_____
iv. other workers - subdued polish colors only; no chips or cracks	_____	_____
v. nails in good repair without sharp corners or edges	_____	_____
d. posture, body mechanics	_____	_____
e. oral hygiene, teeth, breath	_____	_____
f. proper diet	_____	_____
g. care of feet	_____	_____
h. proper footwear	_____	_____
5. Dress code, uniform	_____	_____
a. name/identification badge	_____	_____
b. gait/transfer belt required part of nursing uniform	_____	_____
c. no visible tattoos	_____	_____
d. two small stud-type pierced earrings may be worn; no other visible piercings	_____	_____
e. wedding ring, watch, medical alert jewelry only may be worn	_____	_____
f. no personal communication devices or personal phone calls when on duty	_____	_____

Curriculum	Date	Instructor Initials
C. Lifting and moving residents/heavy objects		
1. Rules for body mechanics	____	_____
2. Safe lifting techniques	____	_____
3. Assistance from other personnel	____	_____
4. Gait/transfer belts	____	_____
5. Mechanical lifts	____	_____
6. Other techniques, adjunctive devices, lift team	____	_____
D. Residents		
1. Overview of the normal aging process	____	_____
2. Types of residents	____	_____
a. geriatric	____	_____
b. mental retardation/developmental disability	____	_____
c. blind, severely vision-impaired	____	_____
d. deaf, hard of hearing	____	_____
e. physical disabilities and deformities	____	_____
f. mental health problems	____	_____
g. Alzheimer's, cognitive impairment	____	_____
i. providing services to residents with cognitive impairment	____	_____
ii. modifying your behavior in response to the resident	____	_____
iii. respect, treating residents as adults	____	_____
iv. person-centered, individualized care	____	_____
v. listen to residents, relate to their reality (not your own)	____	_____
h. young and middle aged residents	____	_____
i. this is the peer group of most employees; maintain professional relationships	____	_____
ii. recognizing manipulation and signs of unhealthy relationships	____	_____
3. Losses, effects of losses on mood and behavior	____	_____
4. Meeting residents' needs	____	_____
a. effects of unmet needs on mood and behavior	____	_____
5. Promoting independence to the extent possible	____	_____
a. giving residents control, allowing them to direct care and make choices	____	_____
6. The Golden Rule	____	_____
7. The Platinum Rule[1]	____	_____
8. Other	____	_____

Curriculum	Date	Instructor Initials
E. Residents' rights		
1. Dignity	_____	_____
2. Rights as a citizen	_____	_____
3. Resident's knowledge of his/her condition and diagnoses	_____	_____
4. Privacy	_____	_____
5. Confidentiality of personal and medical information	_____	_____
6. Freedom from abuse, neglect, misappropriation of property	_____	_____
7. Abuse, neglect, and mandatory reporting procedures	_____	_____
8. Freedom from restraint and involuntary seclusion	_____	_____
9. Personal belongings and property rights	_____	_____
10. Management of financial affairs	_____	_____
11. Rights of association and communication	_____	_____
12. Participation in activities	_____	_____
a. activities for enjoyment and relaxation	_____	_____
b. activities for self-esteem	_____	_____
c. activities for personal empowerment	_____	_____
d. activities for helping others, personal fulfillment	_____	_____
e. reality orientation only if part of plan of care; avoid arguing with residents' reality	_____	_____
f. cognitive enhancement	_____	_____
g. validation	_____	_____
h. reminiscence	_____	_____
13. Advance notice of transfer or discharge	_____	_____
14. Available services	_____	_____
15. Resident volunteer program	_____	_____
16. Right to refuse services	_____	_____
a. responsibility of staff to explain consequences of refusal	_____	_____
b. managing refusals in cognitively impaired residents	_____	_____
F. Terminally ill residents		
1. Right to formulate an advance directive	_____	_____
2. The living will	_____	_____
3. Durable power of attorney/health care proxy	_____	_____
4. Procedures for witnessing or revoking advance directives	_____	_____
5. DNR orders, policies, and procedures	_____	_____
a. managing emergencies (such as choking) in light of a DNR order or living will	_____	_____
b. how to identify residents with DNR orders	_____	_____
6. How to identify residents who should be resuscitated in the event of cardiac arrest	_____	_____
7. Services to families of terminally ill residents	_____	_____
8. Signs of approaching death	_____	_____
9. Policies and procedures for care after death	_____	_____
G. Family dynamics		
1. Family Dynamics	_____	_____
2. Family is an extension of the resident	_____	_____
3. Family adjustments during the transition from home to the long term care facility	_____	_____
4. Family emotions (guilt, fear, anger, uncertainty, sadness, helplessness, overwhelmed, worry)	_____	_____
5. Interacting with families	_____	_____
6. Providing information to families	_____	_____
7. Developing warm, trusting, but professional relationships with families	_____	_____

Curriculum	Date	Instructor Initials
H. Infection control program		
1. Chain of infection	___	_____
a. breaking one link prevents spread of infection	___	_____
2. Spread of germs	___	_____
3. Control of germs	___	_____
4. Handwashing procedure	___	_____
5. When alcohol hand cleaner may be used	___	_____
6. Standard precautions in all departments	___	_____
7. Applying and removing personal protective equipment (PPE)	___	_____
a. preventing environmental contamination with gloves and PPE	___	_____
8. How to inventory, maintain, and discard PPE	___	_____
9. Define biohazardous waste	___	_____
a. proper methods for disposing of biohazardous waste	___	_____
10. Insect and rodent sightings and control	___	_____
11. Signs and symptoms of infection	___	_____
12. Transmission-based precautions	___	_____
13. Importance of maintaining immunizations	___	_____
a. annual influenza vaccine	___	_____
14. Annual tuberculin testing	___	_____
I. Exposure control plan		
1. HIV/HBV/HCV	___	_____
a. mode(s) of transmission	___	_____
b. methods of prevention	___	_____
c. behaviors associated with transmission that are illegal	___	_____
d. current laws and regulations concerning rights of infected individuals	___	_____
e. behaviors related to substance abuse	___	_____
2. Location of the OSHA Bloodborne Pathogen Standard	___	_____
a. explanation of epidemiology and signs and symptoms of bloodborne diseases	___	_____
b. modes of transmission for bloodborne pathogens	___	_____
3. Recognition of tasks and other activities that may involve bloodborne pathogen exposure	___	_____
4. Use and limitations of methods for reducing exposure, including engineering controls, work practices, and personal protective equipment	___	_____
5. Types, use, location, handling, removal, and decontamination of PPE	___	_____
6. Explanation of basis for selection of PPE	___	_____
7. Explanation of biohazard signs, color-coding, and labels	___	_____
8. Action to take, persons to contact, and procedures to follow after potential exposure to blood or other potentially infectious material	___	_____
9. Reporting exposure incidents	___	_____
10. Post-exposure evaluation and monitoring	___	_____
a. medical follow-up	___	_____
11. Information and availability of hepatitis B vaccine, including safety, efficacy, method of administration, benefits of vaccine	___	_____
12. Work-related injuries	___	_____
a. policies and procedures	___	_____
b. reporting an injury	___	_____
13. Personal illness, infection	___	_____
a. attendance policies	___	_____
b. notifying the facility	___	_____

Curriculum	Date	Instructor Initials
J. Safety		
1. Fire and disaster	_____	_____
a. fire, fire drills, procedures to follow	_____	_____
b. tornado	_____	_____
c. hurricane	_____	_____
d. flood	_____	_____
e. ice, snow, inclement weather	_____	_____
f. potential bioterrorism event	_____	_____
g. chemical/hazardous materials emergency	_____	_____
h. bomb threat/explosion	_____	_____
i. earthquake	_____	_____
j. other geographically-specific disasters	_____	_____
k. loss of utilities (power, water, food, heat, etc.)	_____	_____
l. care of medical records, medications, notifications to make	_____	_____
m. residents using oxygen, ventilators, medical equipment	_____	_____
n. emergency generator, identifying generator outlets (plugs)	_____	_____
o. need for facility evacuation, evacuation procedures	_____	_____
2. Code words used for fire, disaster, and emergencies	_____	_____
K. Disaster preparedness/procedures to follow/employee duties		
1. Disaster plan - written and role rehearsal	_____	_____
2. Emergency evacuation plan - written and role rehearsal	_____	_____
3. Major causes of long-term care facility fires	_____	_____
a. unsupervised smoking	_____	_____
b. laundry/dryer fires	_____	_____
c. kitchen/dietary fires	_____	_____
d. electrical fires	_____	_____
e. arson	_____	_____
f. hazardous chemicals	_____	_____
g. extension cords, unsafe outlets, appliances	_____	_____
4. Fire drill responsibilities	_____	_____
5. Location of evacuation plans	_____	_____
6. Location of alarms/pull stations	_____	_____
7. Fire extinguishers, locations ad how to use	_____	_____
8. Fire safety features (doors close, sprinklers, etc.)	_____	_____
9. Fire panel	_____	_____
10. Exterior safety features (fire lane, hydrants)	_____	_____
L. Other potential emergencies		
1. Intruder in facility	_____	_____
2. Violent individuals	_____	_____
3. Drug holdup	_____	_____
4. Concealed handguns, laws	_____	_____
5. Door security	_____	_____
6. Policy and procedures for locking outside doors, admitting individuals after hours . . .	_____	_____
7. Responsibility for identifying strangers in facility	_____	_____
M. Other safety issues		
1. Facility safety committee	_____	_____
2. Safety rules, policies, procedures	_____	_____
3. All employees are responsible for safety	_____	_____
4. Equipment on same side of hallway	_____	_____
5. Avoid blocking exit doors	_____	_____
6. Exit signs, hallway egress	_____	_____
7. Hot water safety	_____	_____
8. Beds and resident care equipment in good repair	_____	_____
9. Wet floors	_____	_____
10. Accident prevention and safety	_____	_____

Curriculum	Date	Instructor Initials
N. Reporting maintenance items/issues		
1. Broken/inoperative equipment	_____	_____
2. Building repairs	_____	_____
a. doors and hardware	_____	_____
b. windows, screens	_____	_____
c. light bulbs	_____	_____
d. holes in walls	_____	_____
e. maintenance log book and work orders	_____	_____
f. preventive maintenance	_____	_____
g. other	_____	_____
O. Lockout/tagout		
1. Policies and procedures	_____	_____
2. Purpose and hazards of energy-isolating devices (locks)	_____	_____
a. recognition of applicable energy sources	_____	_____
b. means of isolating energy sources	_____	_____
3. Who is authorized to apply/remove locks and tags	_____	_____
P. Hazard Communication		
1. Right to know policies and procedures	_____	_____
2. Physical and health risks of chemicals	_____	_____
3. Methods of chemical exposure (inhalation, absorption through skin, etc.)	_____	_____
4. How to determine presence of hazardous chemicals	_____	_____
5. How to reduce exposure risks	_____	_____
6. Location of MSDS sheets	_____	_____
7. How to use MSDS	_____	_____
Q. Resident identification policies and procedures		
1. Wandering resident policies and procedures	_____	_____
2. Wandering resident identification	_____	_____
3. Policies and procedures for door alarms	_____	_____
4. Use of wander system	_____	_____
5. Responsibility for monitoring wanderers	_____	_____
6. Documentation of monitoring and supervision	_____	_____
7. Other facility-specific information	_____	_____
R. Fall risk management		
1. Fall risk policies and procedures	_____	_____
2. Fall risk resident identification	_____	_____
3. Dangers and mortality associated with hip fracture in the elderly	_____	_____
4. Risks associated with head injuries	_____	_____
a. observations to make and report to nurse	_____	_____
5. Responsibilities of all staff related to monitoring residents at fall risk	_____	_____
6. Fall risk reduction measures	_____	_____
7. Importance of maintaining sufficient fluid intake	_____	_____
8. Procedures to follow in the event a resident falls	_____	_____
9. Falls and injury reporting to the state survey agency	_____	_____
10. Importance of proper wheelchair size and fit	_____	_____
11. Use of restraints and alternatives (least restrictive measure)	_____	_____
12. Dangers associated with climbing over/through side rails	_____	_____
13. Importance of locked brakes and small front wheel position during transfers into/out of wheelchair	_____	_____
14. Importance of shoes that are appropriate for floor surface	_____	_____
15. Falls and the quality assurance program	_____	_____
16. Facility commitment to safety and fall prevention	_____	_____

Curriculum	Date	Instructor Initials
S. Emergency actions		
1. Basic first aid procedures	____	____
2. Choking procedure	____	____
3. Maintaining the airway	____	____
4. Need for CPR certification	____	____
5. Breaking a fall	____	____
T. Communications, observation, and reporting		
1. Incidents in long-term care facilities	____	____
a. definition	____	____
b. examples of incidents	____	____
2. Employee incidents	____	____
3. Resident incidents	____	____
4. Visitor incidents	____	____
5. Other types of incidents	____	____
6. Procedures for reporting incidents/accidents	____	____
a. importance of reporting	____	____
b. what to expect after report is made	____	____
c. how to report through the chain of command	____	____
d. procedure for written reports	____	____
e. procedure for witness statements	____	____
7. Quality assurance committee review of incidents	____	____
8. Post incident follow-up and monitoring	____	____
9. Random drug testing following employee incidents	____	____
U. Theft and/or diversions of drugs and/or supplies		
1. Promptly notify your supervisor of suspected theft or diversion	____	____
2. If supervisor is not available notify charge nurse, director of nursing, or administrator	____	____
V. Communications		
1. Employee to employee	____	____
2. Employee to resident	____	____
3. Employee to families and other visitors	____	____
4. Employee to other departments	____	____
5. Employee to visitors from outside agencies	____	____
W. Legal Issues		
1. Scope of practice for your job description	____	____
2. Definition of *standard of care*	____	____
a. importance of meeting and applying applicable standards	____	____
b. why following policies and procedures is essential	____	____
3. Residents and professional boundaries	____	____
a. risks and consequences for boundary violations	____	____
4. Maintaining confidentiality of facility business (salaries, staffing, problems, etc.)	____	____
a. consequences of disclosing confidential facility information to others	____	____

Skills	Date	Instructor Initials
X. The employee:		
1. Can locate and identify the department/facility policy and procedure manual	____	____
2. Describes the proper procedure for reporting absenteeism	____	____
3. Can locate his/her work schedule	____	____
4. Describes scheduling policies, procedures, and responsibilities	____	____
5. Can identify and describe methods of handling resident confusion and anger	____	____
6. Understands how and when to provide emotional support	____	____
7. Can define professional boundaries, how to maintain professional relationships, and list the potential consequences of boundary violations[2]	____	____
8. Demonstrates correct handwashing procedure	____	____
a. Can identify times when hands must be washed	____	____
9. Describes when alcohol-based hand cleaner is appropriately used	____	____
a. Demonstrates how to use alcohol-based hand cleaner	____	____
10. Identifies proper procedures for reporting inoperative equipment and building issues needing repair	____	____
11. Demonstrates good body mechanics for lifting and moving	____	____
12. Can identify abuse, neglect, misappropriation of property, diversion of drugs and supplies	____	____
a. describes reporting requirements	____	____
13. Can locate emergency plans and explain his/her responsibilities in an emergency, external or internal disaster	____	____
a. knows code words for various emergencies	____	____
14. Identifies emergency exits	____	____
15. Identifies potential incidents and accidents	____	____
a. describes how to report incidents and accidents	____	____
16. Identifies residents who wander and understands his/her responsibilities for monitoring	____	____
17. Identifies residents at risk for falls and describes his/her responsibilities	____	____
18. Demonstrates or describes appropriate actions for:		
a. basic first aid procedures	____	____
b. maintaining the airway	____	____
c. caring for a resident who is choking	____	____
d. breaking a fall	____	____
Y. Other content:	____	____
	____	____
	____	____
	____	____
	____	____
	____	____
	____	____
	____	____
	____	____
Z. Notes/Comments:		

Signatures	
Signature of instructor:	Date:
Signature of instructor:	Date:
Employee signature:	Date:

FIGURE A.8

Performance Management Program
Development Outcomes Action Plan

Employee Name: _____

Objective #1: _____

Action Steps: **Completion Date:**

1. _____   _____

2. _____   _____

3. _____   _____

4. _____   _____

Objective #2: _____

Action Steps: **Completion Date:**

1. _____   _____

2. _____   _____

3. _____   _____

4. _____   _____

Objective #3: _____

Action Steps: **Completion Date:**

1. _____   _____

2. _____   _____

3. _____   _____

4. _____   _____

Above are my prioritized development outcomes for the upcoming review period and the specific steps I plan to take to achieve them.

Signature: _____**Date:** _____

FIGURE A.9

QA & A AUDIT

Subject of audit: _____

OBRA REQUIREMENT NUMBER (§_____)

TAG NUMBER(S): F_____, F_____, F_____,
F_____, F_____, F_____, F_____, F_____, F_____,

QUALITY INDICATORS:

1. Administrative rules and regulations

2. Provision of staff and services to residents by those within and outside the facility

DATE:

DATE COMPLETED:

RESIDENT/SAMPLE SIZE:

SOURCES OF INFORMATION:

1. Investigation of compliance with laws and professional standards
2. Investigation of qualifications and services furnished by outside providers
3. Medical record review
4. Systems review
5. Direct observation
6. Other _____

QUALITY ACTION TEAM MEMBERS:

1. Administrator
2. Director of Nursing
3. Infection Control Nurse
4. Nurse Manager and/or Quality Improvement Coordinator
5. Representative from outside provider
6. Other: _____

_____

Response Codes	Yes=X	No=0	Not Applicable =									
Criteria							Resident Number					
	1	2	3	4	5	6	7	8	9	10		
I.												
II.												
III.												
IV.												
V.												
VI.												
VII.												
VIII.												
IX.												
X.												
XI.												
XII.												
XIV.												
XV.												

Response Codes	Yes=X	No=0	Not Applicable =										
Criteria			Resident Number										
	1	2	3	4	5	6	7	8	9	10			
XVI.													
XVII.													
XVIII.													
XIX.													
XX.													
XXI.													
XXII.													
XXIII.													
XXIV.													
XXV.													
XXVI.													
XXVII.													
XXVIII.													
XXIX.													
XXX.													

SUMMARY OF RESULTS OF AUDIT:

Problems/deficiencies identified: _____

Reasons for problems: _____

Actions planned or taken: _____

Correction of problems or deficiencies: _____

Alternatives or revisions of procedure: _____

FIGURE A.10

RESTORATIVE NURSING AUDIT

OBRA REQUIREMENT

TAG NUMBER(S): F221, F222, F282, F309, F310, F311, F315, F316, F317, F406, F498

QUALITY INDICATORS:

1. Specialized restorative nursing care provided
2. Expected outcomes of restorative nursing care

DATE INITIATED:

DATE COMPLETED:

RESIDENT/SAMPLE SIZE:

SOURCES OF INFORMATION:

1. Review of facility policy and procedures
2. Medical record review
3. Interview of residents/staff
4. Observation of residents for maintenance or improvement

QUALITY ACTION TEAM MEMBERS:

1. Quality Improvement Coordinator or Nurse Manager
2. Restorative Nurse
3. Restorative Nursing Assistant
4. Nursing Assistant
5. Licensed Therapist
6. Resident

Response Codes Yes = X No = 0 Not Applicable = #										
Criteria — Resident Number										
	1	2	3	4	5	6	7	8	9	10
I. All nursing personnel are trained in restorative nursing										
A. Nursing personnel understand the restorative nursing philosophy of preventing declines, maintaining and improving residents										
II. The nursing process is used to develop and maintain restorative programs										
III. A licensed nurse oversees the restorative program										
A. The licensed nurse regularly assesses restorative needs										
B. The licensed nurse develops or coordinates the development of restorative nursing programs										
C. Residents restorative needs are assessed on admission for baseline ability/disability										
IV. Restorative services, including goals are listed on the care plan										
A. Specific restorative approaches are listed on the care plan to direct staff in resident care needs										
VI. Restorative services are provided each time the resident requires them.										
VII. Restorative services are provided 24 hours daily to residents who require them:										
A. Range of motion										

Response Codes	Yes = X	No = 0	Not Applicable = #									
Criteria			Resident Number									
	1	2	3	4	5	6	7	8	9	10		

Criteria	1	2	3	4	5	6	7	8	9	10
B. Ambulation										
C. Bowel and bladder management										
D. Bowel and bladder retraining										
E. Activities of daily living										
F. Other										
VIII. Restorative services are documented daily when delivered										
IX. The restorative nurse documents a weekly/monthly summary of progress										
X. The licensed nurse reassesses resident needs quarterly, or as often as necessary to ensure restorative programs are up to date										

SUMMARY OF RESULTS OF AUDIT:

Problems/deficiencies identified:_____

_____

Reasons for problems:_____

_____

Actions planned or taken:_____

_____

Correction of problems or deficiencies:_____

_____

Alternatives or revisions of procedure:_____

_____

FIGURE A.11

REPORT OF
NURSING STAFF DIRECTLY RESPONSIBLE
FOR RESIDENT CARE

DATE: _____

SHIFT	RN		LPN		CNA	
	People	Hours	People	Hours	People	Hours
DAY						
EVENING						
NIGHT						

RESIDENT CENSUS: _____

Daily posting of this information is required for nursing homes participating in Medicare and Medicaid.

FIGURE A.12

_____ AUDIT

OBRA REQUIREMENT

DATE:

TAG NUMBER(S):

DATE COMPLETED:

QUALITY INDICATORS:

RESIDENT/SAMPLE SIZE:

SOURCES OF INFORMATION:

QUALITY ACTION TEAM MEMBERS:

Response Codes	Yes=X	No=0	Not Applicable =									
Criteria						Resident Number						
	1	2	3	4	5	6	7	8	9	10		

Response Codes	Yes=X	No=0			Not Applicable =						
Criteria					Resident Number						
	1	2	3	4	5	6	7	8	9	10

SUMMARY OF RESULTS OF AUDIT:

Problems/deficiencies identified: _____

_____

_____

_____

_____

Reasons for problems: _____

___

_____

_____

Actions planned or taken: _____

_____

_____

_____

_____

Correction of problems or deficiencies: _____

_____

_____

Alternatives or revisions of procedure: _____

_____

_____

FIGURE A.13

Thinning the active medical record

Thinning charts

Nursing personnel are often required to "thin" active medical records to fit in the charts. Forms that have been removed are sent to the medical records department, where they are maintained in each resident's permanent file.

Certain forms must remain on the open chart permanently, whereas others may be removed and filed after a period of time. The listing below provides facilities with guidelines for thinning their open charts.

Common chart form*	Thinning guideline**
Identification and Admission Documentation	
Admission Record/Facesheet	Current Facesheet
Pre-admission Screening (PASARR)	Permanent
Preadmission Assessment/Intake	Three months after admission
Admission Agreement	Financial/Administrative file
Admission Consent	Permanent
History and physical and hospital records	
H&P	Most current
Hospital discharge summary	Most current

Hospital transfer form	Last hospital stay
Other hospital records	Retain pertinent records for three months after hospitalization and then thin
Immunization records	Permanent

Advance directives/legal documents

CPR Directive	Most current
Resident Self Determination Act Acknowledgement	Most current
Living will	Most current
Advance directive	Most current
Durable power of attorney	Most current
Guardianship/Conservator	Most current
Legal incapacitation	Most current
Consents, acknowledgements	Most current
(For example, physical restraints consent, admission consents, consent to treat, consent to photograph, MDS consent, MDS acknowledgement, release of information consent, release of responsibility/leave of absence)	

Clinical assessments (At a minimum, retain most recent assessment plus one previous)

Nursing assessment	Six months to one year

Wound and skin assessments	Six months to one year
Fall assessment	Six months to one year
Bowel and bladder assessment	Six months to one year
Pain assessment	Six months to one year
Mini-mental/cognitive exam	Six months to one year
Restraint assessment	Six months to one year

Minimum data set and care plan

MDS	15 months readily available
Care plan	Current care plan
Specialty care plans i.e.: hospice/dialysis	Current plan
Care plan signature records (if used)	Current plan
Care plan recap (if used)	Current plan

Physicians orders

Computerized recaps or renewals	Three months
Telephone orders	Three months
Interim orders	Three months
Protocols or standing order policies (if used)	Current
Fax orders	Three months

Physician and professional progress notes/consults

Physician progress notes	One year
Cumulative problem/diagnosis list	Most recent

Annual exams	Most recent
Other specialists/consultation	One year
Dental progress notes/exams	One year
Podiatry progress notes/exams	One year
Psychological evaluation	Current

Nursing notes/interdisciplinary notes

Nursing notes or	Three months
Interdisciplinary notes	Six months (excludes quarterly assessments)
Nursing summary forms/flowsheets	Three months

Medication, treatment, and other flowsheets

Monthly medication and treatment records	Three months
Vitals sign record	One year
Weights record	One year
Intake and output records	Three months
Behavior monitoring records	Three months
Other flow sheets (diabetic site rotation, etc)	Three months
Pharmacist/Drug reviews recommendations	One year

Lab, x-rays, and special reports

Lab reports (frequently ordered)	Three months

Annual or interim lab reports	One year
X-ray reports	One year
Special diagnostic tests	One year

Rehabilitative therapy (PT, OT, SLP)

Therapy evaluation	Most recent
Therapy certification/recertification	Three months
Progress notes	Three months
Discharge summary	Most recent
Therapy screen	Most recent

*Once therapy is discontinued thin therapy information for that discipline except the evaluation and discharge summary.

Rehab nursing

Rehab screen	Most recent
Rehab or restorative nursing assessment	Most recent
Progress notes/treatment records	Three months

Social Service, dietary (nutrition services), and activities (therapeutic recreation)

History	Permanent
Progress notes	Six months to one year
Assessments	Most recent

Miscellaneous

Clothing list or inventory list (If required)   Most current

Common chart forms: The chart forms and location are not meant to represent a recommended chart order or forms. Chart order and the types of forms used are facility-specific. This list describes common forms used for documentation found in a long term care record.

** *Thinning guidelines:* These guidelines are recommendations and provide a baseline. Each facility should adapt and develop thinning guidelines that meet the needs of their residents and staff.